Narrative in Healt

Narrative in Health Care
HEALING PATIENTS, PRACTITIONERS, PROFESSION, AND COMMUNITY

JOHN D ENGEL PhD
Scientific Director and Founding Fellow
Institute for Professionalism Inquiry
Summa Health System
Professor Emeritus of Behavioral Sciences
Northeastern Ohio Universities College of Medicine

JOSEPH ZARCONI MD
Vice President for Medical Education and Research
Executive Director and Founding Fellow
Institute for Professionalism Inquiry
Summa Health System
Associate Dean for Clinical Education
Northeastern Ohio Universities College of Medicine

LURA L PETHTEL MEd
Research Coordinator and Founding Fellow
Institute for Professionalism Inquiry
Summa Health System

and

SALLY A MISSIMI RN, PhD
Director of Medical Education and Founding Fellow
Institute for Professionalism Inquiry
Summa Health System

Foreword by

RITA CHARON MD, PhD
Professor of Clinical Medicine
Director of the Program in Narrative Medicine
College of Physicians and Surgeons of Columbia University

Radcliffe Publishing
Oxford • New York

Radcliffe Publishing Ltd
18 Marcham Road
Abingdon
Oxon OX14 1AA
United Kingdom

www.radcliffe-oxford.com
Electronic catalogue and worldwide online ordering facility.

British Library Cataloguing in Publication Data

A catalogue record for this book is available from the British Library.

ISBN-13: 978 184619 193 0

Typeset by Pindar New Zealand, Auckland, New Zealand
Printed and bound by Hobbs the Printers, Southampton, Hampshire, UK

Contents

Foreword

Reading *Narrative in Health Care: Healing Patients, Practitioners, Profession, and Community* is a consequential act, reshaping its reader's fundamental views on health care and challenging basic assumptions about what health care is for. The design of the book is coy, its early sedate presentation of self as a scholarly account of work from many intellectual disciplines acting as a cover for a subversive invitation to radical change. The arguments include not only logically positioned assertions leading to conclusions, but also affectively compelling representations of patients' and clinicians' situations that themselves speak toward conclusions. Both the book's design and the nature of its arguments project, in homunculus fashion, the *form* of the field that it seeks to represent.

Narrative medicine – which has come to include narrative nursing, narrative oncology, narrative social work, narrative pediatrics, narrative psychiatry, and the like – has developed an identity already in its short life. In North America and abroad, clinicians of many disciplines are being summoned to a practice that recognizes patients by receiving their accounts of self. A practice of narrative health care appreciates that the stories of patients and clinicians are at the heart of their work, guiding diagnosis and treatment, providing the foundation for intersubjective relation, guiding ethical discernment and decision reaching, and preserving the sturdy affiliations that occur as a result of hearing and being heard. Such a practice accepts the unity of body and self and with it the duty to heed and hail both. The unity extends from the patient to the clinician in such a practice, for the dividends of reflective narrative practice are interior consonance for both patient and clinician.

In the Program in Narrative Medicine at Columbia University, where the concept and the name arose in 2000, health care professionals of many disciplines are joined by patients and family caregivers to develop narrative skills. Through their training in close reading, attentive listening, and reflective writing, they find themselves achieving effective alliances as a consequence of their shared narrative work. It seems as if recognition generates recognition, so that the ill person seen in a clearer light is able to see the seer in a clearer light. This spiral extends throughout the life of this clinical dyad, resulting in increasingly accurate diagnostic impressions and clinical treatment for the patient, and ever more deeply satisfying self-becoming for the clinician.

The concepts and theories presented and propounded in this book have concrete clinical sequelae. Office routines are turned on their heads as nurses and doctors simply say to patients, "Tell me what you think I should know about your situation." The clinical notes that record transactions with patients look different by virtue of increased narrative skill – higher word-to-number ratio, longer stretches of ordinary language, affectively dense tone, and even the occasional use of the word "I." Patients are apt to be invited to read these accounts by their authors, if only as a check of the text's accuracy (in effect, we show what we write to patients, asking them "Did I get it right?", and elevating them to the status of authority which they should have occupied all this time but never did). Clinicians write about their patients in new genres, as the reader of this book learns from the many poems and stories written by nurses, doctors, social workers, and students reproduced here. Patients are encouraged to write about their own perspectives on illness, and so the sick person and the one caring for that person are both given more robust evidence on which to base their clinical conclusions.

The authors of *Narrative in Health Care: Healing Patients, Practitioners, Profession, and Community* – a social scientist, a physician/executive, a counselor, and a nurse – are the engineers of a shift in culture, curriculum, and practice at Summa Health System, a large mid-western health system affiliated with the Northeastern Ohio Universities College of Medicine. Starting from different positions, the four authors have converged in a strong and shared commitment to narrative health care. They conceptualize narrative health care practices within frameworks derived from the social sciences and psychology, and, to a lesser degree, phenomenology and autobiographical theory. They relate the development of narrative medicine to relationship-centered care, patient-centered care, and complex responsive processes of relating theory, positing that narrative medicine can help clinicians to develop the skills required to practice relationship-centered care. The narrative skills that they deem salient to effective health care are reading and telling complex stories, reasoning with stories, writing reflectively, compassionate presence, mindful listening, practicing empathy, and exercising the moral imagination. This book details – with exercises, resource texts, and abundant scholarly apparatus – how each one of these can be developed and strengthened. The authors rehearse evidence that narrative practice is good both for patients and for clinicians, and they offer arguments that the risks entailed in *not* using these methods routinely in practice are significant.

By the time a clinician has finished reading the entire book, he or she has lived through something of moment and is no longer able to return to the self that pre-dated the reading. As I absorbed chapter after chapter, I found myself changing state, perhaps to the sublime. I found myself welling with ideas and epiphanies and memories and plans, feeling at the same time excited, perplexed, contrary, and proud. These are the kind of ideas that gradually break on one, much like the sunrise or sunset. Over a natural period of time – the rise, the set, the journeys on the A train reading a chapter or two a day – the whole picture changes gradually in color and brightness and pattern and beauty, until the viewer simply cannot remember what it was like before its transformation.

The vision to which we are granted access by the authors recognizes the congress among many disparate species –patients, doctors, nurses, social scientists, psychologists, phenomenologists, literary scholars, and chaplains. When three of the four authors worked with my faculty and me in a Narrative Medicine Workshop at Columbia recently, they enacted the deep work of which they are capable. What became evident to us and the other workshop participants were the dividends of their longitudinal collaboration – the gradual nearing in and clarifying of perspective, the almost sibling familiarity shared among them, the utter respect with which they handled one another's ideas, and the freedoms visited on each of them by virtue of the recognitions by the others. In this book they are, in effect, generously sharing with the rest of us what they have personally learned from their own narrative medicine – that when chasms are bridged and when mutual recognition occurs, the persons of groups grow in insight, collegial respect, and power, coming to know things that none of them could have known alone.

There are some things that this book cannot accomplish. For example, there is very little literary theory in this work. None of the authors is trained in literary studies, and so the book adds little to our disciplinary understandings of how narratology and literariness might illuminate the clinical situation, or what the clinical situation can reveal to the literary scholar. The fact that there are some things which this book does *not* do adds to my sense of its importance, because it suggests that there are many dimensions or facets to narrative medicine, and that interrogating each of them may be able to deepen our current understanding of the field.

I find this book to be a meta-phenomenon as well as a text. That is to say, its very *existence* means something. If it were written in invisible ink, it would still exert an influence on health care, because its having been written by writers other than the ones who initially proposed the model demonstrates that there is now a coherent discipline of narrative medicine or narrative health care whose roots can be traced, whose intellectual antecedents can be identified, and whose sibling ways of thinking can be named. The meta-textual aspects of the book treat the field as if it were a natural state of affairs such as one finds in biology – the Sargasso Sea, perhaps, or a *Volvox* colony, or a thyroid gland. The interested observer watches how this entity moves, how it eats, how it touches others, how it matures, who its nearest relatives are, and how widely spread it has become. This is an uncanny proof that the thing itself exists.

Finally, I foresee that this work will change health care. Because of its scholarly rigor, its multi-voiced sources, and its highly practical features (lists, activities, key ideas and key references, and primary texts written by health care professionals and patients), this work will be a guide in the field for those who practice medicine or nursing or social work. The book *establishes* that there is a field to be practiced, a need to practice it, and a means to develop the wherewithal to do so. Let us hope that its readers see the sun rise on a new day in health for us all.

Rita Charon MD, PhD
April 2008

About the Authors

John D Engel PhD

John, a social scientist, is Scientific Director of the Institute for Professionalism Inquiry, Summa Health System, and Professor Emeritus of Behavioral Science at the Northeastern Ohio Universities College of Medicine. His research interests are the philosophy of social science inquiry, qualitative methodology, narrative health care, and integrating humanities and social sciences with health professions education and practice and care of the dying. John served as founding associate editor for *Qualitative Health Research* and edited the methodology section of that journal. He has been a member of the Editorial Board of *Evaluation and the Health Professions* since its inception. He has published extensively in his areas of interest, and is currently engaged in conducting a longitudinal study of professional development as well as a participatory action project on the impact of narrative practice in a department of family medicine.

Joseph Zarconi MD

Joseph is Vice President for Medical Education and Research at Summa Health System, and serves as Executive Director for Summa's Institute for Professionalism Inquiry. He is Professor of Internal Medicine and Associate Dean for Clinical Education at the Northeastern Ohio Universities College of Medicine. A practicing nephrologist, he is active in the teaching of medical students and residents on nephrologic topics as well as in the areas of virtue ethics, narrative ethics, narrative medicine, and professionalism in medicine.

Lura L Pethtel MEd

Lura is one of the four co-founders of the Institute for Professionalism Inquiry, Summa Health System, and coordinates research and evaluation activities as well as the *Humanism and Healing Arts* conference series. Lura is co-leader and teacher in the narrative medicine course for family medicine residents at the Summa Health System, and conducts research in the ecology of medical careers. During her long tenure at the Northeastern Ohio Universities College of Medicine, she served as Associate Dean and taught in the areas of behavioral sciences and humanities, and co-directed courses in spirituality and medicine and end-of-life care. For the Last Acts organization she authored a training program for spiritual companions for the dying.

Sally A Missimi RN, PhD
Sally practiced critical care nursing for 10 years, and is currently Director of Medical Education at Summa Health System. Her interests include health system organizational culture, narrative health care, and the effects of the introduction of humanistic practice on hospital culture. Sally is also actively involved in developing health care career pathways for inner-city middle and high school students.

Acknowledgements

In addition to our many patients and students to whom we have dedicated this work, we also express deep gratitude to our mentors, colleagues, and friends who have taught us about the human condition and how it is transacted and represented through stories. We have been inspired by their generosity in sharing with us the most intimate details of what it means to suffer with an illness, to develop as professionals, to be responsible for others, and to live a moral life.

The scholarship of two people in particular, Rita Charon and Trisha Greenhalgh, has stimulated our thinking about and understanding of the place of narrative in health care.

We are deeply indebted to the many people who have supported us in the development of this work. The following individuals read earlier drafts of portions of this book, and provided important and meaningful feedback: Jack Coulehan, Paul Durbin, Thomas Inui, Martin Kohn, John Thomas, and Peter Ways. We are especially grateful to the following people who gave most generously of their time and provided comments on the majority of chapters: Rita Charon, Richard Frankel, Deborah Jones, and Anton Kuzel.

Responsibility for any misunderstandings and/or errors resides with us alone.

To our patients who have honored us through their invitations into their narratives. And to our students, who give us hope that through narrative work, health care can be a moral and healing community.

Introduction

Once upon a time those who were sick spoke to those who sought to heal about the intimate details of their bodies and their lives. Healers had little else to offer other than their personhood. They were present to witness the suffering of others and to humbly care for the bodies and spirits of those others and, in so doing, they cared for their own spirits as well. However, as this art of intimate connection was slowly and inevitably influenced by sociocultural and economic trends as well as advances in technology and scientific knowledge – knowledge about the interior space and workings of the human body – encounters between the sick and their healers became more influenced by various forms of mechanical and therapeutic technology. The biophysical condition of patients certainly benefited from these advances. However, with these benefits came the moral and spiritual separation between patient and healer and a devaluing of the intimate narratives that took place between them. In the healer's well-motivated enthusiasm to cure, a dramatic imbalance evolved between practice framed by biophysical medicine and practice centered on caring and actively listening to the patient's story. Although not all of the current dissatisfactions between patients and practitioners can be attributed to this imbalance, we believe that what matters most to patients and practitioners is the connection that obtains through the sharing and honoring of complex illness narratives. We believe that the same is true of the stories that are shared among practitioners about who they are and what it means to care for others.

We come to these beliefs through the particular pathways that each of our careers has taken in medical education and clinical practice. We represent four separate but related disciplines within the health care enterprise – social science (*JDE*), medicine (*JZ*), counseling (*LLP*) and nursing (*SAM*). All of us are educators with varied experiences across all levels of medical education. We would like to share with you events that brought us to the belief that narrative practice is critical to health care.

JOHN (*JDE*)

In the late 1970s, I had the opportunity to lead a project that was to reconfigure third-year clinical education for medical students at a large mid-western medical school. One of my colleagues, an internist who taught on the wards, invited me to spend a few days with him as he conducted patient rounds with the students. As I spent the next several days with him, I was most struck by the variety of stories that were exchanged and the power that they had to either heal or dehumanize. This experience preceded a narrative turn in the social sciences and the professions. Although I did not have an intellectual framework (a disciplinary language) to discern the phenomenon as narrative and to understand the nuances between it and communication, it was clear to me that the stories which I witnessed mattered to patients, physicians, and students. Moreover, the transaction of stories had an impact along a moral continuum from "good" to "bad." I understood in a rather naive way that both patients and physicians seemed satisfied when the practitioner worked with the patient to tell his or her story, and did so in a respectful and attentive way.

The outcome of encounters seemed much more problematic when the patient's story was either dealt with in a superficial manner or not solicited at all. I remember in particular one senior resident who whirled into a patient's room and, without acknowledging the person in the bed, briskly drew back the sheet covering the patient, pressed on the abdomen and said to the health care team assembled at the end of the bed, "Well, he's OK to discharge today." And turning back to the patient, the resident said "We'll turn you back into a human being today", and then left with the team following in tow. I was the last person to leave the room, and as I reached the door I turned to see the patient crying and asking me "What do I do now?" By lunchtime the story of this encounter had spread among the students on the medical service and, as I sat having lunch with several of them and listening to them talk about the encounter, it struck me that some thought the encounter was unprofessional (although they didn't use that word), and others represented it as just another "overworked" and "burnt-out" resident. Regardless of the particular interpretation of the event, it seemed to me that the story had power to dehumanize the patient and influence young medical students' perceptions of their profession, and to both disempower and dehumanize the resident as a health care practitioner. Since that time I have been witnessing and collecting stories that are transacted in health care settings, and trying to make sense of their ubiquity and their power to heal and damage patient and practitioner as well as the community of practice.

JOSEPH (*JZ*)

After a year or two of teaching principles-based ethics to third-year medical students as their clerkship director – teaching that I found increasingly and painfully boring – a faculty colleague and medical humanities scholar, Martin Kohn, offered an alternative approach, introducing me to the field of narrative ethics. We shifted our approach of teaching ethics in the context of autonomy, beneficence, non-maleficence and justice, to seeking out ethical dilemmas as they arose in particular patient stories – stories in which our students had participated. Since that time, we have engaged students in the writing of these stories, and in sharing them in small group discussions. Each student is asked to identify from among her assigned patients one whose experiences have created for her some degree of "moral turbulence" – that sense of queasiness one feels when something in the patient's experience is particularly troubling. The student writes in the patient's voice in an attempt to capture what she imagines to be the patient's "interior monologue." The student is encouraged to depict in this writing the patient's lived experience of illness. These stories are then shared and discussed in our group meetings.

These sessions continue to be some of the most powerful experiences of my professional life. They are often emotional. Students cry, they challenge each other, and they expose their innermost selves in a safe space. Reflecting on their stories in these meetings and on my own experiences with patients continues to remind me of why I went down this road to medical work. I have learned that while the students believe that they are writing about their patients, most of what they write is, in fact, about themselves – who they are as young professionals, what they stand for, and how they hope to *be* as doctors. These are aspects of their own professional identity development that they come to discover simply by being in their patients' narratives.

In the early years of this work, one student wrote himself into the patient's story as riding into his hospital room on a white horse. This student was depicting himself as a hero – not from the perspective of being above the patient, more powerful, or more pure, but in the sense of possessing some special characteristics consistent with the hero myth. Many times since, students have depicted themselves on this white horse in more figurative ways. This powerful and recurrent theme in our students' writing has caused me to ponder the urgency with which students want to help their patients, and to rescue them from their distress. And they see themselves, among all members of the caregiving team, atop the white horse, perhaps because they are the ones who get to spend more time with the patients. They connect with patients in ways that too many interns, residents, and attending physicians have often long since abandoned. They seek to know who their patients are, to understand their life experiences, hopes and dreams, and to operate in their narratives. As a medical educator, it is clear to me that as these students proceed into internship, residency, and practice, many of them will, as a result of their educational experiences, get down off these white horses and never remount them. Much is lost when that occurs. My continued interest in teaching students and young physicians an appreciation of the power of narrative medicine is, I suspect, a way of trying to keep them on their steeds, for all of our sakes.

LURA (*LLP*)

Several years ago, I was doing my rounds as a pastoral care volunteer in the intensive-care unit (ICU). I am not a chaplain. I am a counselor, an educator and a compassionate-care volunteer. Over several days, I had become acquainted with the niece of a patient who occupied the first bed inside the unit. Apart from an elderly brother, this woman was the patient's only other relative, and she and her aunt were very close – like daughter and mother, she explained. The patient had progressed very satisfactorily, and in fact she was going to be discharged home the next morning.

As I began my rounds early the next day there was obvious activity surrounding the aunt's bed – the "crash team", a nurse said. Soon the attending physician, several residents and nurses exited the area, all looking sober, and silently they pulled the curtain around the bed. The attending physician, recognizing me and knowing my role in the ICU, came over to me and said, "She died unexpectedly just a short while ago. We don't know why and we couldn't bring her back. We were going to send her home this morning. We expect her niece to arrive soon – will you be here when she comes?" As I looked around the area I saw each member of the team now standing or sitting alone or perched on the edge of a table, all at different spots, separated, motionless, and silent.

Shortly afterwards the niece and her uncle, the patient's brother, arrived, and as they were about to peek inside the curtains, I quickly walked over to them. I held them outside the curtains, hoping that some member of the team would come to the niece's side. Not one of them moved. The residents seemed to have moved even further from the scene, the nurses were busily engaged elsewhere, and the attending physician had disappeared. As best I could, I explained what had so suddenly occurred. When they seemed to understand, I took the niece and her uncle inside the curtains to be with the patient for a while. As the niece sobbed and kissed and stroked her aunt's cheeks, she brokenly related that she had called the unit earlier that morning and talked to her aunt, and had brought the articles from home that she wanted. They were in the bag she was clutching. Her uncle was voiceless, the tears quietly sliding down his cheeks.

When they were ready to leave, I walked with them out of the doors and into the hallway, thinking that I would accompany them to their car. (I must insert here that the niece was morbidly obese and quite tall, and I am fairly slight in stature and weight.) As we began to move slowly down the hallway, the niece, still sobbing, began to hyperventilate severely. There was no place to sit down, and as I struggled to hold her upright, I feared that she would pass out. She would surely fall on me. Her uncle was very frail and still silent, not really grasping what was happening. A doctor whom I didn't recognize passed us in the hallway and said "Everything okay?" as he continued on. Finally, I caught sight of a chair just inside the door of a room close by. I managed to guide the niece to the chair, which was almost too small for her girth, and knelt down beside her so that I could command her attention and quiet her breathing. Eventually she uttered a few words: "I came to take her home. Why did she die?"

This incident will forever remain poignant in my memory, and it has raised many questions that I have struggled with over the years. What was happening to these *professional* caregivers when all of their medical knowledge and technology failed them? Where was the caring? Where was the compassion and empathy? Where was the spiritual connection to the individuals in their keep? Were they paralyzed emotionally or were they struggling to detach from their emotions? Were they allowing some sense of failure and guilt to override their sense of honor to their chosen profession and to their patients? This event, among the many others that I have witnessed in clinical environments (not all as unfortunate as this one) clearly emphasizes for me the true significance of narrative medicine which lies at the very heart of relationship-centered care. The everyday work of medicine is fraught with difficult moments, yet still demands intimate narrative connection with patients and families, regardless of the particular surprises or outcomes.

SALLY (SAM)

A typical afternoon in the coronary care unit (CCU) where I worked brought patients who waited out the days hoping that their chest pain would disappear, but were ultimately admitted when their hopes never materialized. One such afternoon brought a call from the emergency room with a report of the admission of a 65-year-old woman who had experienced day-long chest pain and who had arrived at her physician's office with symptoms suggesting an impending myocardial infarction (MI). When an ambulance was called, she refused transport even after the seriousness of her condition had been emphasized numerous times. She promised her doctor that she would go directly to the emergency room, which was less than a mile away from the office. She wanted to drive herself and not leave her car. The physician agreed to allow her to drive, and called the emergency-room staff to notify them of her imminent arrival.

When the physician arrived in the CCU after completion of his office hours, the patient had still not arrived. Calls to her home went unanswered. The unit was not busy – in fact, she would be one of only two patients if she ever arrived. Eventually she did turn up, over four hours after her initial office visit, and she was sent directly to the CCU. A quick assessment noted that she had in fact suffered an MI, and the CCU team descended on her with all the known interventions and treatments available to minimize the damage.

As the team worked with the patient, the physician became increasingly agitated as he noted the passing of the evening. At one point he walked into the room and asked the patient why it had taken so long for her to get there, and didn't she know that she had been jeopardizing her health and wasting his time while he waited for her. She responded in a very weak and tired voice, saying that she had to clean the kitchen, do a few other things, and get pizza before she could go to the hospital. The physician responded by yelling at her, calling her stupid and inconsiderate, and stormed out of the room barking orders to the resident to "follow up on this one", because he was leaving.

The team was also surprised at her response, many of them, including myself, muttering about her stupidity. How could she be so ignorant of her condition? Why would she spend so much time doing "things", including getting a pizza? What were her priorities?

I took a break from the unit long enough to run to the cafeteria to pick up food for the staff, none of whom had eaten during the entire shift. As I walked past the waiting room, I saw a gathering of people – an older man in a wheelchair, a younger man talking with an obvious speech disability, another woman who was taking care of three small babies, all dressed in old, ill-fitting clothing too thin to keep them warm in the harsh winter weather. They were gathered around a small table eating pizza! I stood in the hallway, absorbing the scene, realizing that I was watching this family eat a meal provided by my patient. This was her family – her priority.

Life's priorities are personal, as evidenced by this patient's story. This collection of souls gathered in the waiting room, huddled over a pizza, was her family – the people who contributed to her unique identity. And even at the expense of her own life, she took care of them. I understood, for the first time that evening and probably for the first time in my nursing career, the importance of the patient's perspective, the patient's story, and her lifeworld.

At the time when this story unfolded, I could not identify narrative health care as a term, let alone as any theoretical basis for discussion around what a person's story meant to her understanding of illness. However, I did understand clearly how patients construct their illness stories in the context of their life stories – what is important to them, not to me. I also learned a valuable lesson about assumptions and priorities. Both are extremely personal and powerful in their influence over how we see the world and how we act on what we know about the world.

Although we all come to the importance of stories in different ways, we share a strong belief that the practice of health care and the education of health care professionals at all levels ought to honor the narrative character of clinical work. It is that belief which motivates and informs our thoughts in this book.

At the start, we should say a few words about our understanding of the terms *narrative* and *story*, since they form the core of this work. Factions within various disciplines that are concerned with narrative hold differing viewpoints about these terms or ideas. Some who do theoretical work in the field argue for a difference between the terms *narrative* and *story*. Others who are more practice-oriented tend to treat the terms interchangeably. Our pragmatic bent leads us to the latter position. We understand narrative to be a story – written or oral – where a teller motivated by unexpected events describes to a recipient of the story a sequence of purposeful actions with a plot (a beginning, middle, and end) set in a particular context and arranged according to a temporal structure. It is the inter-subjective nature of the dialogue in encounters between patients and health care practitioners and among practitioners that constitutes a fundamentally communicative act – a narrative.

We are interested in non-fictional narratives, often told in the first person and occurring in four related situations – patient and practitioner encounters, the practitioner reflecting on self, practitioners engaging with other practitioners and profession about work, and practitioners engaging with community members. One of our aims is to show how narratives that occur in these situations inform important micro- and macro-questions that frame, sometimes silently, today's health care contexts. Across the pages of this book, we consider questions such as the following.

- How can we provide authentic care for patients in the midst of medicine's current moral crisis? How do mindful listening and co-creation of illness stories provide therapeutic sustenance for both patient and practitioner?
- How can health care practitioners renew themselves and affirm their intentions for entering practice?
- How can we reaffirm professionalism through community?
- In the current climate, what ought to be the character of biomedical ethics, professionalism, and social responsibility?

Our second aim is to illustrate how to enhance narrative skills that contribute to narratively competent practice in the four situations noted above.

We also need to be clear that throughout this book our main focus is on narrative transactions among patients and health care practitioners who, in the main, have both the capacity and the motivation to be honest and trustworthy in their relationships. We do not treat in any serious fashion special circumstances in which people are intentionally deceptive about the stories that they author. And we do not deal with special issues that obtain with narratives in mental health situations. Such theoretical and practical matters are certainly important, but remain outside the boundary of our current work.

Finally, underlying our writing is a vision of patients who suffer with a wide variety and degree of chronic diseases. We also envision patients who seek more than technological "fixes" and detached encounters with their caregivers. This vision is based on our experience and belief that chronic illness represents a majority of conditions that bring together patients and their caregivers. This is not to say that narrative health care does not have merit in situations that are acute or emergent, and for encounters that are brief and amenable to a predominantly biomedical approach. Any practitioner will encounter patients who, within and across encounters, prefer, want, or need a variety of relationships. The skills of narrative practice enable practitioners to intuit appropriate boundaries for each encounter and nurture the wisdom to act in consort with their patients for their mutual benefit.

Part 1 of the book consists of three chapters that describe the historical context and theoretical foundations of narrative health care. They contain the most abstract material in the book, and perhaps also the most intellectually challenging for those who are unfamiliar with these foundations. We believe that a familiarity with the arguments in these first three chapters will allow you to decide, in practical and informed ways, why and how to engage narratively with patients, colleagues, and members of your community.

Chapter 1 rehearses the development of modern medicine and shows how clinical thinking and practice are connected to larger movements in the history of science in such a way as to create the legacy of biomedicine and the counter-revolutions to this dominant form of thinking both inside and outside of medicine. In Chapter 2 we describe one of these counter-revolutions, namely the turn to narrative in certain academic disciplines as well as particular professions. In this chapter we take up the issue of the narrative representation of illness, life stories, and personal identity. Here there is an important focus on the narrative structure of clinical practice within the patient–practitioner relationship. Part 1 concludes with a chapter that more fully examines the nature of the patient–practitioner relationship and how narrative health care and the practitioner's narrative competence frame the character of this relationship.

In Part 2 we consider the place of narrative in four health care situations – patient and practitioner, practitioner and self, practitioner and colleagues/profession, and practitioner and community. In each situation, the power and utility of story to enable one to better understand who one is and what is transacted in complex encounters are examined and illustrated. Two of these situations are framed within the central notions of caring in Chapter 4. We show how patients present their problems to health care practitioners as rich and complex stories. We argue that health care practitioners need to function within their patients' stories and, with the patients, to reconstruct new story lines that bring understanding and relief of suffering. Furthermore, we argue that when health care practitioners take time to reflect on themselves, their practices, and their personal lives, they engage with patients and others in a more healthful manner. The other two situations are framed within a broader social organization of colleagues and communities in Chapter 5. In this chapter we discuss narratives of professionalism – stories of what it means to be a professional and how the sharing of these narratives serves to form both a collective and individual sense of professional responsibility. We suggest how these narratives influence individual practitioner behavior and the collective development of medical education.

Following the material of Chapters 1 to 5, we have placed an Interlude – a play that two of us (*LLP* and *JDE*) have adapted from Leo Tolstoy's novella, *The Death of Ivan Ilyich*. This play is an example of "readers' theater", and serves two functions in this book. First, we want to bring this profound piece of literature to those who may not have had the opportunity to enjoy its rich texture and critical moral deliberation. Secondly, readers' theater is an important vehicle for nurturing a variety of narrative skills that are discussed in Chapter 6.

We view Part 3 of the book as the core of our project. New skills are needed to live and practice in today's health care environments. A new or revitalized narrative competence in conjunction with scientific competence is required for a fulfilling practice of health care. Six narrative skills are examined in Chapter 6, and the relation of these skills to clinical work is highlighted. We also provide illustrations of reflective writings connected to clinical encounters. This chapter describes and illustrates the following skills:

1 practicing compassionate presence and mindful listening
2 exercising moral imagination and expressing clinical empathy
3 reading and interpreting complex texts
4 writing reflectively and telling complex clinical stories
5 reasoning with stories
6 engaging in narrative ethics.

You have the opportunity to practice some of these skills through several narrative stretching exercises. Chapter 7 discusses the effects of narrative success and the risks of non-narrative practice. We explore the evidence for successfully using narrative skills in clinical transactions, and the risks of not doing so, both for the practitioner and the patient.

In Chapter 8, in Part 4, we offer a number of conversations with health care practitioners (nurses and physicians) who reflect upon the character, impact, and future of narrative health care.

The weight of the arguments that we have constructed in this book is clearly on the side of advocacy for a reflective and nuanced narrative practice by health care professionals. That said, we want to be clear at the outset that we have framed our remarks while cognizant of the few empirical studies that have examined how physicians decide to relate to patients (1), and patient reports of their preferences about physician communication styles (2, 3). These initial studies suggest to us that both practitioners and patients place dynamic boundaries around the styles of interaction which they prefer at a given time. We believe that these boundaries are contingent on practice contexts for practitioners and health/illness contexts for patients. Collectively, these studies suggest that the primary care physicians who were studied view a substantial number of patient encounters as *routine*, where a biomedical model is useful, and even preferred (1). And patient preference studies suggest that approximately one-third of the patients in the studies preferred a biomedical style in their physicians (2, 3). In thinking about these studies and their limitations, it seems to us short-sighted to interpret these preliminary results as evidence against widespread training and practice in narrative care, as some have done. We hope that this narrow point, namely that some patients under certain circumstances seek a biomedical encounter, will not be over-generalized. It is, we believe, more productive to view these studies as nuance and contingency in clinical relationships wherein a majority of patients prefer a more relationship-centered form of care, and a significant number of patient encounters are judged by practitioners to require more relationship-centered and narrative care. Thus it is our position that prudent practice requires health care practitioners to reflect wisely on the boundaries of engagement in caring for particular patients, and to be skillful in multiple contingent ways of relating with their patients.

We wish to note that we have followed certain conventions in writing this book. Each chapter begins with a table of contents and key ideas. Each chapter concludes with suggestions for further activities. We have used the terms *health care practitioner, clinician, caregiver,* and *medical professional* to represent physicians, nurses, allied health professionals, counselors, and clinical psychologists. We deviate from this convention only when the content is specific to a single profession. We find awkward the use of he/she or s/he to represent the impersonal pronoun. Consequently, we use "she" in all cases except where an accurate representation of the situation requires otherwise. The reference to "she" is not restricted to a person of that gender. When illustrating material from our personal lives, we have indicated the particular person by using initials in italics. Where patient names are used, we have used fictitious names. Finally, we have provided a glossary of terms at the end of the book.

We invite you to join this emerging field of narrative health care by considering the arguments that we offer in these pages. Moreover, we encourage you to share narrative teaching exercises as well as stories of your own experiences with patients and colleagues that contribute to the growing list of important narratives. You can do so by logging on to www.summahealth.org and then in the "Find It" box, type "Institute for Professionalism Inquiry" and post your ideas.

REFERENCES

1 Miller WL. Routine, ceremony, or drama: an exploratory field study of the primary care clinical encounter. *J Fam Pract.* 1992; **34**: 289–96.

2 Swenson SL, Buell S, Zettler P *et al.* Patient-centered communication: do patients really care? *J Gen Intern Med.* 2004; **19**: 1069–79.

3 Swenson SL, Zettler P, Lo B. 'She gave it her best shot right away': patient experiences of biomedical and patient-centered communication. *Patient Educ Couns.* 2005; **61**: 200–11.

PART 1

Historical Context, Genealogy, and Current Viewpoints

In this first part of the book, we examine the historical background that sets the stage for the place of narrative in the theory and practice of medicine. We travel back to the seventeenth century to rehearse the importance of Enlightenment thinking for the evolution of science, and then move gingerly through the eighteenth and nineteenth centuries to inspect the movement of science into the education of health care practitioners and their resulting practice. We then describe what many have referred to as a *narrative turn* in several disciplines and professions. This leads us to a discussion of the place of story in current models of the patient–practitioner relationship. These initial chapters contain the most abstract and theoretical material of the book. One could access other parts and chapters of the book without considering this material and still understand the content. However, we encourage readers to consider the arguments of Part 1 so that they can apply the content of the remaining chapters to their practice in an informed way, rather than as simply another "technology" for practice.

CHAPTER 1

Medicine, Medical Practice, and Knowledge

There is . . . no essential medicine. No medicine that is independent of historical context. No timeless and place-less quiddity called medicine.

Arthur Kleinman (1: 23)

. . . the doctor, by virtue of accepting science so totally, creates a total imbalance, forgetting the art of healing, forgetting the art of engagement, forgetting the art of listening, forgetting the art of caring and ceasing to invest time with the patient. So I believe that medicine has lost its human face.

Bernard Lown (2: 1)

- A CLINICAL STORY
- THE MAKING OF MODERN MEDICINE
- SCIENCE, PARADIGMS, AND MEDICINE
- THE LEGACY OF BIOMEDICAL MEDICINE
- BIOMEDICINE: COMPETING VIEWPOINTS

KEY IDEAS

- Practices and values of modern medicine have their foundation in the social and intellectual contexts of the mid-nineteenth century.
- US medicine during the nineteenth century was heavily influenced by Scottish and French clinical medicine and German medical science.
- US physicians returning from training in Germany believed that science was the key to medical progress as well as reforms in medical education.
- Medicine embraced a form of seventeenth-century science built upon the work of Bacon, Descartes, and Newton, and based on empirical observation, material mechanisms, reductionism, determinism, and dualism.
- This seventeenth-century paradigm evolved into the dominant system of thought that propelled future medical scientists and physicians to act as objective observers striving to eliminate subjective features of their practices.
- This stance laid the foundation for a biophysical approach to the patient.
- Biomedicine fosters an approach to suffering that values increasing levels of abstraction and distance from the lived experience of the sufferer – an approach that is abstract, context free, and impersonal.
- The critique of biomedicine strives to reconnect mind with body and return the patient as a reflecting and reflexive self to the center of the clinical relationship.

A CLINICAL STORY

"Get ready to listen to his complaining", I had told the medical student assigned to the nephrology service that month. His left hand was now so awkward, the patient would tell us over and over again, ever since the surgery. He was an otherwise fairly active 58-year-old African-American man whose longstanding poorly controlled hypertension had damaged his kidneys irreparably. In preparation for the eventual hemodialysis treatments that would keep him alive, I had referred him to a vascular surgeon. He would need an arteriovenous fistula – a surgically created connection between the artery and vein in his wrist – so that the artery's high-pressure, high-flow circulation would be diverted into one of the veins draining the hand. That surge of blood flow would, over a number of weeks to months, allow the vein to blossom into a very large and tough blood vessel from which the blood, through large needles, could be delivered to the artificial kidney and filtered in the dialysis process.

Sometimes this alteration of the blood supply to the hand can harm the tiny nerves which activate the functions of the hand. Occasionally the neurologic impact is quite disabling, but more often the consequences are subtle and clinically insignificant.

So it was, it seemed to me, in this man's case. Despite his unrelenting bemoaning of the post-operative results, no significant dysfunction could be detected by my careful objective neurologic examination. More importantly, I argued, the "little bit of clumsiness" that so upset him was on his left, non-dominant hand, after all. I was incredulous at his persistence, and what seemed to me to be the whining of a man who failed to appreciate that I was offering him life-saving treatments designed to add years to his life. The fact that he was incapable of seeing this "bigger picture" had actually begun to annoy me.

During this hospitalization for an unrelated problem, he continued to focus our attention on his "ruined" hand. He could not be consoled by our pointing out that his hand clearly appeared to be acceptably functional by our examinations. So when the medical student joined the team, I felt the need to prepare him for my patient's perseverations. "Get ready to listen to his complaining", I had instructed.

Three days into the hospital stay, outside of his room, I was reviewing his progress with the residents on the team in anticipation of his discharge. One of the residents jokingly asked whether I thought it was safe to discharge him with such a significant disability in his hand. Would he be able to care for himself? How would he take his medicines? Perhaps we should consider nursing home placement. They, too, were fatigued by the chorus of his complaining. As the chuckling waned, the medical student came out of the patient's room. The question he then asked me is one which continues to haunt me. "Did you know", he queried, "that this patient is a pianist?"

As every physician does throughout a career, I presume, I carry certain patients with me, in the pockets of my white coat. These are patients who, for better or for worse, have transformed me through my experiences with them for all of my subsequent medical work. This man is one such patient, one for whom I have never forgiven myself.

I am inclined to believe that had I been aware of this man's piano playing, and furthermore of how important it was to him, I would have encouraged him to consider methods of dialysis that would have allowed him to avoid such a disabling operation on his arm. Had I made assumptions about this man, assumptions which grew from my own biases, my own ignorance? The life I was offering him was a compromised one, and it was a compromise that didn't have to be. This patient and his medical student remind me of the importance of heeding one's own advice. "Get ready to listen to his complaining", I had warned.

JZ

This is not an atypical story of an encounter between a patient and a doctor. What is remarkable about the encounter is the coexistence of two stories – the doctor's and the patient's story – one dominant and active, the other silent and passive. What accounts for the different character of these stories? Why is one story privileged over the other? What is the outcome of this situation for both patient and doctor? What does each person bring to the telling of and listening to the patient's story that influences their interpretations?

One way to understand what transpired between patient and doctor is to examine the intellectual and social contexts of the tasks which this doctor brings to the encounter. The physician needs to gather information about the patient's condition in order to provide care. In this encounter, there exists the possibility of attending to multiple forms of knowledge in performing those tasks, including the biophysical information gained from the medical history, physical exam and laboratory tests, the patient's story of his lived experience with a less than fully functional hand, and the meaning of that condition for his sense of self. In this encounter, one kind and source of information is valued over another. Biophysical information, perceived as "objective" and coming from physical touch and laboratory data, screams while information perceived as "subjective", the patient's illness story (his experience of suffering), is silenced. Why does the clinician, seeking to serve the best interests of the patient, perform in this manner? To examine these questions we look to the historical and social contexts which frame the development of the physician's profession and the conduct of his actions.

THE MAKING OF MODERN MEDICINE

We begin with a brief look at the rise of the medical profession in the USA. Others have carefully documented and interpreted this history, and for our purposes we need only rehearse the highlights of their arguments (1–5). We rely on the excellent original work of Paul Starr, Kenneth Ludmerer, Roy Porter, and Helen Dingwall for our story of this period. We recognize that within any given period there are multiple and often competing idea systems at play. In this chapter we try to represent the dominant patterns of thought. Readers who are interested in this complex history are encouraged to examine the materials listed in the "Further Activities" section at the end of the chapter.

The establishment and ascendance of any profession is the outcome of a struggle for cultural authority and upward social mobility. In speaking about this phenomenon with respect to the medical profession, the historian Paul Starr (3) suggests that professional movements are explained by factors internal to the profession, such as practitioners' ability to generate new knowledge, and their personal and economic ambitions, and factors external to the profession, namely broad changes in culture and society. For our purposes, we bracket the period from the eighteenth through to the early twentieth century, a particularly important period for the formation of the medical profession. During this period, forms of medical education within the profession and concurrent social events external to medicine serve as the backdrop for the development of the profession and professional practice.

From the late 1700s through to the early 1900s, the relationship among the characteristics of medical education, the profound influences of Scottish, English, and French clinical medicine and German medical science, and the reform of American universities became important as the formative context for the clinical case that begins this chapter.* During this period, doctors in the USA were trained by apprenticeship, by attending one of the several dozen proprietary medical schools, or in some instances by both. Originally created as a supplement to apprenticeship, the proprietary school consisted of two 4-month periods of classroom instruction during the winter months, with the two terms being exactly the same in content – anatomy, physiology, pathology, chemistry, medical jurisprudence, theory and practice of medicine, principles and practices of surgery, obstetrics, and diseases of women and children. There were no written examinations to be passed, and scientific subjects received little, if any, attention. Everyone was graduated.

Americans who had the money furthered their medical education in Europe. In the late eighteenth century, several notable residents of Philadelphia, such as John Redman, John Morgan, William Shipper, and the politically influential Benjamin Rush (referred to as the "founding father" of American medicine) trained at the University of Edinburgh. Edinburgh, and to a lesser extent Glasgow and Aberdeen, was an intellectual "hotbed" of the European Enlightenment. In the early years of the Scottish enlightenment, Edinburgh was a particularly unique center of intellectual activity. A very special pattern of cultural values linked with local institutions was evolving that, unlike other intellectual and political circles, addressed the whole of mankind. Scottish scholars were broadly trained in numerous disciplines. Consequently, they approached and studied any particular phenomenon from multiple perspectives. For the theory and practice of medicine, these attitudes and values manifested themselves in close observation of patients, written recording of observations, an appreciation of the patient's story, and case-based clinical training in the classroom and local infirmaries. The Philadelphia physicians who studied in Edinburgh during the early years of the Scottish Enlightenment brought these experiences home and transformed them into their practices and teaching (6–8).†

Later, in the first half of the nineteenth century, Americans usually studied in Paris, since France had become the center of medicine of that period. In fact, American medicine through the time of the Civil War predominantly reflected the French model of medicine. For two generations, French clinicians inspired physicians everywhere by developing an understanding of modern pathology and physical diagnosis, the application of statistical techniques to clinical

---

* Certainly there were other factors that influenced American medicine. Doctors in colonial America tried to emulate medical forms typical of eighteenth-century England as a model. However, as Starr (3) notes, because of cultural and social class differences between the two countries, the English model did not transfer. Readers who are interested in the development of medicine in Britain should consult C Lawrence's book *Medicine in the Making of Modern Britain 1700–1920* (London: Routledge; 1994).

† The Scottish Enlightenment held the seeds of its demise. The early years were strongly opposed to Baconian inductivism and reductionism. However, the interdisciplinary openness and tolerance and broad education of its scholars, which had brought rapid intellectual expansion and innovation, was increasingly replaced by specialization and reductionism as scholars sought to firm up their disciplinary boundaries and expertise.

research, and the focused use of the hospital as the primary vehicle for teaching and anatomic pathology, having learned the importance of the educational link from the Scottish system. French physicians such as Laennec transformed the structural practice and teaching of medicine.

Laennec's invention of the stethoscope in 1816 revealed a new range of clinical information, linking signs and symptoms with anatomic pathology. His invention conjoined technology and medical practice forever (9). Like most technology it was both used and misused. In 1848, the Harvard physician, essayist, and poet, Oliver Wendell Holmes (10: 25), penned the following pointed poem.

The Stethoscope Song: a professional ballad

There was a young man in Boston town,
    He bought him a *stethoscope* nice and new,
All mounted and finished and polished down,
    With an ivory cap and a stopper too.

It happened a spider within did crawl,
    And spun him a web of ample size,
Wherein there chanced one day to fall
    A couple of very imprudent flies.

Now being from Paris but recently,
    This fine young man would show his skill;
And so they gave him, his hand to try,
    A hospital patient extremely ill.

Then out his stethoscope he took,
    And on it placed his curious ear;
Mon Dieu! said he, with a knowing look,
    Why, here is a sound that's mighty queer!

There's *empyema* beyond a doubt;
    We'll plunge a *trocar* in his side.
The diagnosis was made out, –
    They tapped the patient; so he died.

Then six young damsels, slight and frail,
    Received this kind young doctor's cares;
They all were getting slim and pale,
    And short of breath on mounting stairs.

They all made rhymes with "sighs" and "skies",
    And loathed their puddings and buttered rolls,
And dieted, much to their friends' surprise,
    On pickles and pencils and chalk and coals.

So fast their little hearts did bound,
 That frightened insects buzzed the more;
So over all their chests he found
 The *rale sifflant* and the *rale sonore*.

He shook his head. There's grave disease –
 I greatly fear you all must die;
A slight *post-mortem*, if you please,
 Surviving friends would gratify.

The six young damsels wept aloud,
 Which so prevailed on six young men
That each his honest love avowed,
 Whereat they all got well again.

This poor young man was all aghast;
 The price of stethoscopes came down;
And so he was reduced at last
 To practice in a country town.

Now use your ears, all that you can,
 But don't forget to mind your eyes.
Or you may be cheated, like this young man,
 By a couple of silly, abnormal flies.

Oliver Wendell Holmes

French physicians worked alongside surgeons in the hospitals and gradually viewed pathology as local rather than generalized pathophysiology. These clinical pathologists, using astute clinical observation alongside pathological anatomy at autopsy, disabused medicine of speculative and monistic theories of disease. The result was a radically different empirically observed classification of disease based on linking two sets of data – signs and symptoms from clinical investigation, and descriptive data from morbid anatomy. Equally important, this movement changed the focus of debate about medical truth from dogmatic assertions based on authority to empirical evidence. These changes were not only an advance in medical knowledge, but also a social transformation in the way that patients were perceived and in how hospitals were organized.

The French clinical method had evolved to include three important features.

- It told clinicians exactly what to do to get the required results – that is, take the patient's history, conduct a physical examination and other investigations.
- It simplified orders.
- It provided criteria for validation – morbid anatomy (11, 12).

However, with this emphasis on connecting clinical observation with anatomical correlation, French physicians neglected the study of basic biological science and exhibited hostility toward experimental laboratory research. Ludmerer (4: 23) notes that these values came from a belief that ". . . medical knowledge resulted from chance clinical observation, not from the manipulation of nature through experimental design." As a result, French medicine had little to say about the root causes of disease, and this made way for another movement in medicine.

By the 1840s, German medical science had reconceptualized its approach so that it emphasized experimental study of biological organisms rather than speculative philosophy. From the mid to late 1800s, German medical scientists developed cell theory, restructured modern physiology, and developed cellular pathology and bacteriology. Unlike their French counterparts, German scientists relied on the laboratory to advance medical knowledge as they emphasized the connection between sciences – biochemistry, physiology, experimental pathology, pharmacology, and bacteriology – and disease and therapeutics. Of course, some French and British workers had also followed experimental medicine and made great advances. However, the key factor in the dominance of the German medical model was the intimate connection between medical research and the German university. German universities had gained dominance in many areas of higher education, including philosophy, social science, linguistics, and natural science. Within the intellectual culture of the university, German medical scientists operated in an environment that valued free thought, flexible organization, and well-equipped laboratories. These ingredients made German medical science the envy of all others.*

The influence of the movements in Scottish, English, French, and German medicine was felt in US medical practices from the mid 1800s to the early 1900s. During the Civil War, severe limitations in the training of US physicians to care for the injured and diseased soldiers became obvious. The training of most physicians had taken place through apprenticeship and proprietary schools, with much smaller numbers having some training in English, Scottish and French schools. Following the Civil War, waves of American physicians intent on increasing their skills started to go abroad to further their training. Given the zeitgeist of reverence for German medicine, many chose to concentrate their studies in German universities. Bonner, quoted by Ludmerer (4), notes that approximately 15,000 American physicians engaged in serious study in Germany, beginning around 1870 and ending in 1914 when German–American relations were suspended because of World War One. Americans who studied in Germany were in general young, well-to-do men from the east coast. When they returned to the USA, these men often became the leading physicians of their generation (4).

---

* It is interesting that this same phenomenon – an intimate connection between medicine and the university as a whole – accounted for the prominence of Scottish medical education in an earlier period (6, 7).

The German university experience of these physicians had two profound developmental effects on medical education and clinical practice in the USA. Returning American physicians believed passionately that the key to medical progress lay in controlled experimentation, and that the hallmark of a successful career lay in intellectual distinction through medical scholarship rather than medical practice. However, most of them were frustrated in their attempts at academic careers and in their desire to emulate their German mentors. From the mid 1800s to the early 1900s, the institutional organization to support high-quality medical research was either weak or lacking altogether. However, following the Civil War, the American university began to grow into its modern form, and by the early twentieth century the university more commonly embraced medicine and the education of physicians. As Ludmerer (4: 39) put it, the American university became ". . . the provider of a secure institutional home, a source of financial support, and a reservoir of intellectual and emotional encouragement." Essentially, this turnabout was connected to the reconstruction of the idea of the university as a place for storing or conserving knowledge. Now, the university was thought to be a place where new information and knowledge were to be generated. It followed from this line of thinking that medicine, like other disciplines, was to produce knowledge through a process of scientific inquiry and would be served well by integration with basic science disciplines. Furthermore, it took special, well-qualified people to learn and teach medicine.

The resulting reform narrative of medical education is well documented, so we represent here only one small part to illustrate the profound structural and organizational change in the profession (4, 5). From around 1870 to 1893, enormous curricular changes were forged with great difficulty at pivotal US medical schools – Harvard University, the University of Pennsylvania, the University of Michigan, and Johns Hopkins University. Charles Eliot, the new president at Harvard University, had been trained as a chemist at that institution. After taking his degree there he studied in France and Germany. His studies abroad had convinced him of the critical importance of science to medicine, and of learning science in the laboratory.

Ludmerer (4: 49) observes that two powerful senior faculty members, Oliver Wendell Holmes and Henry Jacob Bigelow, resisted Eliot's ideas, characterizing them as ". . . faddish glorification of German science and offensive disdain for clinical acumen." In the ensuing conflict, Eliot's views prevailed, and in 1871 a new set of reforms was introduced. While the development of medicine at Johns Hopkins was different, in part because it was a new school and created a curriculum *de novo*, the overall story of these elite schools was one of structural and organizational change. Admission requirements were established, the course was lengthened to four years, compulsory oral and written examinations were instituted, science disciplines (anatomy, physiology, physiological chemistry, pathology, pharmacology, and bacteriology) were placed at the core of the new curriculum, the presence of clinical disciplines increased, and teaching methods emphasized active learning and equal emphasis on laboratory and clinical bedside teaching.

With these reforms, the place of science in medical education and practice was firmly entrenched. Furthermore, being faithful to a prevailing foundational view of knowledge, curriculum developers placed the basic sciences at the earliest stages of medical education. This placement had a powerful effect on the early enculturation of people into the profession. Because of the critical nature of this arrangement, we need to explore the nature of the type of science that laid the foundation for what constituted appropriate knowledge in the clinical disciplines and practice in clinical environments.

SCIENCE, PARADIGMS, AND MEDICINE

If the intimate connection between science and medicine facilitated the reforms for the profession and for professional practice by the end of the nineteenth century, what was the nature of science at that time? What form of science did medicine bring into its house? An understanding of the answers to these questions resides in the historical roots of seventeenth-century science. The work of three seventeenth-century intellectuals had a profound effect on the development of science and medicine up to the beginning of the twentieth century (13, 14). In order to understand these developments, we look to the work of three intellectual giants – Francis Bacon (1561–1626), René Descartes (1596–1650), and Sir Isaac Newton (1642–1727).

Francis Bacon, a philosopher, graduated at the age of 16 years from Trinity College in Cambridge, England. He was inspired by various figures of the Renaissance, and revolted against the prevailing Aristotelian teaching of his time. Although he greatly respected Aristotle, he saw the Aristotelian method as useful only for disputation and contention, and of no help in producing works that would benefit the life of men (15). To rectify the situation, Bacon proposed an inductive method of discovering truth. This method was founded upon empirical observation, analysis of observed data, logical inference resulting in hypotheses, and verification of hypotheses through continued observation and experimentation. The purpose of the method was to enable man to attain mastery over nature and to exploit it for his benefit.

René Descartes, a philosopher and one of the founders of modern epistemology, argued that reality existed in two separate and independent realms – mind and body (16).* He used the metaphor of the machine to describe the body as a series of anatomical parts that functioned without any notion of human mind. This early form of Cartesian dualism was superseded by an epistemological dualism that emphasized two different ways of knowing – subjective awareness and direct observation. This dualism figured prominently

---

* In part, Descartes' position was taken as a means of pursuing science without interference from the church.

22

in the work of nineteenth-century French medicine. As discussed above, the acts of visual inspection and autopsy were the basis of clinical truth, and the patient's subjective account of illness was dismissed as unreliable and irrelevant to physical diagnosis. In the modern era, another form of dualism continues to exist – that of physician as active knower and patient as passive known (17).

Sir Isaac Newton's work on the mathematical principles of the natural world was based on a novel conception of the universe. He postulated that the universe worked like a coherent and materially structured machine with well-oiled, interchangeable parts that produced order and regularity. His ideas further reinforced the idea of the body as a machine in which the whole was merely the sum of the parts. Newton's influence greatly contributed to a growing interest in scientific method. Method as both philosophy and technique is the link between Newton and the emerging disciplinary fields of the period, including medical studies such as physiology.

These three great intellectual projects contributed to the European Enlightenment Age,* the age of reason, and a scientific paradigm based on empirical observation, material mechanisms, reductionism, determinism, and dualism. These ideas had a revolutionary impact on the practice of science and on beliefs and values about what should be the proper domain of medical thinking and practice. Paradigms act as powerful frameworks that influence, both overtly and covertly, how scientists think about and proceed in their practices to uncover knowledge about the world in which we live (18). Equally important, paradigms also discourage and rule out competing ideas of what constitutes proper method and legitimate truth.† Perhaps most critical for our purposes is the fact that paradigms become part of the physician–scientist's cultural background, and the unreflective hold on these thoughts and beliefs runs the risk of having them become dogma.

This seventeenth-century paradigm became a system of thought that normalized what constituted proper scientific work and propelled scientists and physicians in future eras to act as objective observers and to regard nature as independent from themselves and unaffected by their acts of observation. The

---

* The European Enlightenment stretched from the early seventeenth century to the beginning of the nineteenth century. As a cultural and reactionary period, it was distinguished by the passionate efforts of dominant personalities to make *reason* the absolute ruler of human life. It started in Scotland with figures such as Hutcheson, Cullen, Gregory, Block, the Monroe family, Reid, Hume, and Smith. In England, the empiricism of Bacon, Hobbes and Locke flourished. The period was especially nurtured by Scottish, English, French, and German philosophers.

† When communities of scholars use paradigms to function dogmatically and unreflectively as gate-keeping mechanisms, a process of hegemony results. It needs to be recognized that the dogmatic use of paradigms to sanction and legitimize certain forms of inquiry is not behavior exclusive to the dominant scholarly community. There is always another non-dominant community of scholars holding firmly in a dogmatic way to their preferred paradigm. This phenomenon has been referred to as "paradigm wars", and signals both intellectual and moral disagreements about truth and science. As a consequence, there is often a small set of scholars seeking rapprochement between the "warring" factions. The use of dualities often signals this state of affairs – for example, Newtonian physics vs. quantum physics, quantitative vs. qualitative inquiry, generalization vs. specialization, evidenced-based medicine vs. narrative medicine.

philosopher Alfred North Whitehead (19) has described this way of thinking as a connection between an avid interest in detailed facts and a passion for abstraction and generalization, both in the service of capturing knowledge that was universal and certain. McWhinney (12: 18), describing this period, cites Toulmin (20) as saying:

> From 1630 on, the focus of philosophical inquiries has ignored the particular, concrete, timely and local details of everyday human affairs: instead it shifted to a higher, stratospheric place on which nature and ethics conform to abstract, timeless, general and universal theories.
>
> (Toulmin, 1992: 34–5)

Abstraction, along with the decontextualization of particular features of a phenomenon (the separation of subject and object), became hallmarks that were carried into succeeding periods and into the house of medicine.

The significance of the Enlightenment resides in two factors – momentum and commitment to a particular form of practice (13). The momentum resulted in a spectacular array of accomplishments in the natural sciences. These accomplishments convinced others, physicians among them, that commitment to the same methodological principles that had proved so successful in the natural sciences was essential for inquiry in other fields of endeavor. Foss and Rothenberg (13: 28), philosophers of science, note that ". . . the dynamic relationship of reason, defined in terms of method, and the idea of progress come together to influence human activities. The result was nothing short of a revolution in human affairs in general, and among other areas, medicine in particular." Eric Cassell, a physician, notes the character of the "revolution in human affairs" in medicine (21). He argues that medical science, demanding adherence to its rules of conduct, attends only to objects that are value-free, independent from one another, and mechanical in nature (i.e. each part has its specific function). According to this view, functional capacity is dependent on structure, and in order to change function one must effectively alter structure. Thus all aspects of the human condition boil down to explanations in bio-physical-chemical terms. Cassell (21: 188) writes:

> Because of these postulates, medical science could not deal effectively with individuals, value-laden objects, things that change over time, or wholes that are greater than the sum of their parts. Since that list contains the characteristics of persons (*be they patients or doctors*), medical science could not handle persons – but disease lay clearly within its purview. (emphasis added)

The inheritance of this world view is the biomedical model, to which we now turn.

THE LEGACY OF BIOMEDICAL MEDICINE

We have seen that US physicians who trained between the late 1700s and the early 1900s were predominantly influenced by Scottish, English, French, and German medicine, and consequently embraced versions of a natural science paradigm that laid the foundation for a biophysical approach to patients. This approach evolved into what is referred to as the biomedical model. Every theory or model of medicine conceptualizes three dimensions – disease, patient, and therapy. Within the biomedical model, disease is represented as a process of deviations from the norm of quantifiable biological variables. The idea of causes is based on Newton's model of a force operating on a passive object. In biomedicine this idea is manifested in the doctrine of specific etiology – a harmful agent acting on a person to produce a disease. The patient is conceptualized as a passive biological entity made up of parts, the sum of which is a whole human body. Therapy is conceptualized as a physical intervention that neutralizes the harmful agent (13). Thus biomedicine claimed exclusive somatic authority.

Medicine of the nineteenth and twentieth centuries swore allegiance, in effect, to a paradigm based on a seventeenth-century paradigm of classical physics (Newtonian physics). This paradigm's position on what legitimately constitutes reality (ontology) and knowledge/truth (epistemology) very often operates silently and unreflectively within succeeding generations of biomedical researchers and clinical practice. As a result, human phenomena have either been excluded from scientific inquiry or the scientific approach to human conditions has been required to conform to a method of inquiry that mimics what is perceived to be "normal biomedical science." Furthermore, within this paradigm, the concepts that guide inquiry are objectivity, a-historicity, a-culturicity, a-emotionality, and universality.

Many scholars have argued that to follow these principles is a misapplication of the paradigm. As suggested by the physician George Engel (22: 131), "What advocates of the universality of the biomedical paradigm fail to appreciate is that, like its seventeenth-century counterpart in classical physics, the biomedical model represents a limiting case, the utility of which is in no way diminished as long as its use is restricted to the phenomena for which it was designed." And so the failure to recognize this fact in large part accounts for biomedical research that has been insensitive to the interaction of human phenomena such as age, race and gender with physiological and pathophysiological processes. In clinical medicine, it has fostered an approach to suffering that has moved toward increasing levels of abstraction and increasing distance from the lived experience of the sufferer – an approach that is abstract, context free, and impersonal. In fact, in traditional medical education, students are taught to "take histories" when what they are really doing is "creating histories." By turning the patient's complaints into generalizable concepts which can then be categorized explicitly for the purposes of constructing a differential diagnosis, the students make a particular patient's experiences the same as for all who have such experiences.

Several of my colleagues and I were "living with" third-year medical students during their 10-week rotation in internal medicine. Late in the afternoon it was routine practice for one of the senior residents to assemble the house staff, including the students, to conduct ward rounds for patients currently on the service. The patient chart rack would be rolled into the conference room and, while sitting around the table, the resident responsible for the care of a patient would review the chart notes. Sometimes the resident had seen the patient that day and sometimes not! I was struck by the lack of any contact with patients during the almost 90-minute period, and after the session I expressed my curiosity to one of the residents whom I had known as a senior medical student. Her response was that the patient's presence wasn't really necessary because all of the pertinent information was in the chart, diabetes was diabetes, and it saved time not having to talk with a patient who would tell the "same old story" yet again.

JDE

At this point, it may seem that we are arguing against the biomedical model and setting the stage for its rejection, which is not exactly the case. Our position is that the hegemony of the model has resulted from its unexamined or misunderstood limitations as it has been applied to biomedical research, and particularly as it has framed approaches to patient care. Abstraction and generalization clearly have their benefits, and are essential to the successful transactions of our daily lives. However, we do argue that abstraction, as a totalizing approach to human behavior, often suffers from what Whitehead (19) has referred to as the *fallacy of misplaced concreteness* – that is, of mistaking our abstractions for reality. An abstraction is built from the analysis of particulars, and then the resulting concept is used to represent all of those particulars. What is forgotten is that no abstraction can represent fully the details of all of the particulars. Thus abstractions are at best partial truths. This position is representative when applied to human phenomena such as illness. Hypertension or esophageal cancer as abstract disease categories cannot fully represent the illness in a person suffering from the disease, much less in multiple patients suffering from the "same disease." The person with damaged kidneys is not just a person with chronic kidney disease, but a person often suffering from a diminished sense of self-worth. However, within a model of medicine that values only, or even predominantly, the abstraction (because the abstractions are the result of a scientific process that yields the only trustworthy form of knowledge upon which to form therapeutic actions), what is devalued is the lived experience of the patients, and thus their viewpoints are less germane to good clinical care.

The various levels of abstraction for a patient with esophageal cancer are illustrated opposite.

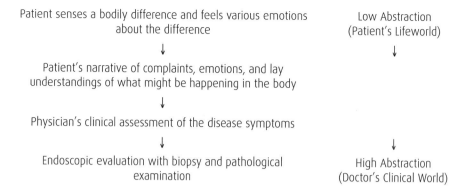

As we move from the patient's lifeworld to the doctor's clinical world, we gain the benefits of abstract clinical diagnosis. A doctor attending exclusively within a biomedical framework risks forgetting the critical nature of a patient's lived experience – the patient's full narrative. When this is the case, the physician's clinical judgment is influenced by a spirit of abstraction (23) and subject to the fallacy of misplaced concreteness. As a result of this behavior, the patient's complaints are disparaged as unimportant and untrustworthy data, in favor of objective truthful information representing the pathology and pathophysiology of the material body. Another, perhaps less dramatic example of this process is the person who has chronic daily headaches but a normal physical exam and a normal MRI, and who is told *"There is nothing wrong with you."* Such an abstract biomedical approach to patient care divides physicians from the particulars of the lived experience of their patients and, as we shall discuss later, divides physicians from themselves as healers. To put it another way, the Enlightenment legacy of what constitutes legitimate knowledge, namely that which comes through science, serves to delegitimize the patient's story and narrative knowledge of the clinical condition.

<u>Misplaced Concreteness</u>

Worship abstractions
Fondly blind what matters most
Me, Myself, and I

JDE

The reliance on medical practice framed within a biomedical model has been criticized in various ways during the latter part of the twentieth century, and more so during the early part of the present century. The criticism has come from within segments of the profession, from patients, and from social science and humanities disciplines connected to medicine. We believe that this criticism is in the service of restoring balance between an approach to the patient that is steeped in the tradition and practice of a biomedical model, and an approach that honors and integrates the mutual influence that physicians and patients have on one another and the substrate of lived experience that provides context and meaning to clinical diagnosis and treatment. As we now turn to this critique, which sets the stage for current movements to reform clinical method, it is important to remember this issue of restoring balance on both sides of the stethoscope.

BIOMEDICINE: COMPETING VIEWPOINTS

Biomedicine, because of its physicalist and positivist assumptions, has achieved an increased understanding of the mechanisms of disease and, consequently, stunning breakthroughs in therapeutic interventions. In this respect, it is easy to understand why Western medicine has rightly been heralded as a modern achievement, second to none. However, in the midst of this success there is a sense of crisis. Patients are often dissatisfied and practitioners too often feel unfulfilled. This situation has stimulated criticism from both within and outside the medical profession. The thrust of the criticism is that biomedicine is simply too narrowly focused in its research as well as its associated clinical practice.

In what follows, we want to emphasize that we see the various critiques as movements that are representative of the discontent expressed by collections of thoughtful individuals. Furthermore, we see these movements as moments of cross-talk among multiple disciplines – moments ripe for the cross-fertilization of ideas. And finally, we believe that these discussions are, at root, what the physician–philosopher Edmund Pellegrino (24: x–xi) has characterized as critical to the development of a philosophy of medicine:

> . . . the nature of the healing relationship; the concepts of health, disease, illness, suffering, death, and dying; the relationship of medical knowledge to knowledge in the sciences, social sciences, and humanities; the phenomena peculiar to clinical judgment; the definition of a patient's good; and the nature of trust and hope in the phenomenology of illness.

Scholarly work on these issues will lead to a general theory of medicine. The ideas embedded in the various critiques and calls for reform, along with their associated assumptions and values, all contribute to the discussion of such a theory.

Although various critiques of biomedicine emanate from particular philosophical and socio-political positions, they are in agreement that the prevailing medical model (theory of medicine) essentially separates mind and body so that the patient has no *self.* For scientific medicine, the object of treatment and cure is a diseased body. All other considerations (e.g. anxiety, pain, discomfort, compassion, care) are relegated, too often in a pejorative manner, to the art of medicine. Thus the general thrust of all of the critiques of biomedicine is to reconnect mind and body and to return the patient as a reflecting and reflexive self to the center stage of clinical care. To indicate the flavor of these critiques, we briefly sketch the arguments of several notable figures whose focus on the limitations of biomedicine comes from different vantage points, and consider different orders of reality.

John Powles (25), speaking from socio-historical and ecological viewpoints, notes that in the area of infectious diseases, a bastion of so-called success for the biomedical model, the greatest benefits to increased health of individuals and communities came early on from influencing man's interactions with the environment – sanitary control, the provision of food, and the regulation of births. Only later did biomedicine contribute by way of immunization and antibiotics. Powles also points out that there is a strong positive relationship between increased ischemic heart disease and increased economic development. His criticism is leveled at the exclusive and hegemonic application of biophysical medicine to increasing health. His strategy is to show the significant and dramatic influence of social and economic factors on the health of individuals.

Arthur Kleinman and his colleagues in the social medicine department at Harvard Medical School have argued that medicine's crisis can, in part, be attributed to biomedicine's exclusive focus on the concept of *disease* (disordered biological processes) to the exclusion of the equally important concept of *illness* (the person's experience of suffering) (1, 26, 27). Kleinman's cross-professional training in medicine and cultural anthropology enables him to view biomedicine as just one cultural form of practice among many. From this perspective, he argues that what is radically different in this form of medicine is its knowledge (epistemological) and reality (ontological) commitments. Biomedicine, he claims, differs from most other forms of medicine in several ways.

- It insists on materialism as the grounds of knowledge.
- It dismisses dialectical modes of thought.
- It requires single causal chains to specify disease etiology as a rationale for specific therapeutic regimens.
- It insists on a conception of nature that excludes the teleological (1).

Through its insistence on the primacy of these factors, biomedicine constrains the practitioner to construct disease as the narrow focus of study and treatment, leaving no room for the patient's experience of suffering. As Kleinman notes, the patient's stories are perceived as subjective self-reports that are untrustworthy, and as such the physician is to reinterpret the illness story in the service of the authentic story of disease as pathology. He goes on to say (1: 32–3):

> The result is a huge split between the constructed object of biomedical cure, which is the dehumanized disease process, and the constructed object of most other healing systems, which is the all-too-humanly narrated pathos and pain and meaning-directed perplexity of the experience of suffering. . . . Nor does any other tradition so distrust and choose not to elaborate nonspecific therapeutic sources of efficacy

that are associated with the rhetorical mobilization of the charismatic powers of the healer–patient relationship that persuade patients and families to believe in successful outcomes and thereby enact scenarios of efficacy . . .

Thus, in Kleinman's view, biomedicine constructs the task of therapeutic work without legitimizing the patient's story of suffering, and in so doing reduces the physician's ability to participate in a mutually healing relationship.*

In 1977, George Engel (28) published an article entitled "The Need for a New Medical Model: A Challenge for Biomedicine" in the journal *Science*. Being a practicing physician, Engel's interest was in advocating a new model for medical practice that brought into focus more than pathophysiology in the therapeutic care of the patient.† He argued for a systems approach to the patient, that would take seriously the interactions of biological, psychological, and social dimensions of disease. Engel's thinking has had its greatest influence among primary care physicians. It has encouraged them to integrate information from a variety of levels and to seriously pursue the emotional and social effects of illness in the care of the person (29).‡

In 1987, at the invitation of Alvin Tarlov, then President of the Henry J Kaiser Family Foundation, 45 prominent and influential physicians, social scientists, and philosophers gathered for a Conference on the Biopsychosocial Concept of Illness and Disease. The focus of the meeting was on the patient–physician relationship and the kind of information necessary for care of the patient, and for training physicians for that care. A number of "white papers" were written and circulated prior to the meeting and then discussed widely during the four-day event. One of the more controversial papers, written from the interests of primary care medicine, was that of Michael Schwartz, a physician, and Osborne Wiggins, a philosopher (30). These scholars argued that a *comprehensive* theory of medicine includes a biomedical concept of science focused on explanation of material processes, and also a phenomenological concept of science focused on understanding the lived body as an extension of a unique concrete individual. They advised a clinical practice that seeks biomedical diagnostic evidence (understanding through causes) that can only be extracted through a phenomenological process – actively engaging the patient's story of illness. This move was meant to restore the patient as an active participant

---

* Physicians who incorporate their humanistic and communication skills into the relationship with patients (and there are many) do so against this dominant portrait of the profession and what it means to be professional.

† The term "biopsychosocial" has been associated with Engel's work. Over the years this label has proved to be off-putting – a piece of jargon that has not necessarily increased understanding of the substance of Engel's work. For too many the model has been reified and contrasted to the "biomedical" model, and thus has perpetuated yet another dualism.

‡ Critics of the model have argued that it encourages physicians to think that they have an "objective" view of patients' psychological and social perspectives, and this sanctions their abuse of power by intervening in people's social lives as well as in their illnesses.

in the relationship, and compensate for the narrowness and insufficiency of biomedical practice in the total care of a suffering person.

One of the most complete discussions of the benefits and limitations of biomedicine has come from Laurence Foss and Kenneth Rothenberg (13). Their sentinel work deserves serious consideration. These scholars use ideas and data from open systems theory, information theory, and artificial intelligence to outline a theory of medicine that they refer to as *infomedicine*. In writing the Foreword to Foss's second book, McWhinney (31: x–xi) summarizes the new model:

> The new paradigm rests on two foundations. First, the view of the human body as a machine is replaced by the view of the body as a self-organizing system. The body has some machine-like features, and medicine can still make progress by working at this level. However, an adaptive, information-processing system, mindfully as well as autonomically interacting with its physical, social and cultural environments, has properties possessed by no machine, including those of self-organization and the capacity for self-transcendence.
>
> The second foundation is the separation of energy from information, each with its own causal mechanism. . . . Energy transfer produces change by action on a passive object . . . information transfer produces change by releasing a process that is already a potential of the system. In the case of the human subject, this potential has a life, and mind, of its own. The resulting change, the physiological response, reflects this life and mind. Hence, in a medical context, health and disease are not biological but psychobiological phenomena.

Unlike the previous alternative viewpoints outlined above, Foss's theory makes a break with dualisms by making biomedicine a limiting case of infomedicine. Such a conceptualization has the potential for revitalizing medicine as both theory and practice.

Finally, we turn to another viewpoint that offers its critique from outside biomedicine and science per se. Beginning in the late 1980s, a number of physicians, literary scholars, and psychologists advanced the view that understanding human behavior is fundamentally a narrative activity, not a science (27, 32–37). The critique by Kathryn Montgomery Hunter, a narratologist, is representative of this literary viewpoint. Her criticism of the form of science represented in biomedical practice is consistent with that rehearsed above. Her alternative view is offered as follows (34: 5):

> Patients' stories within medicine are more or less pared-down autobiographical accounts that chronicle the events of illness and sketch out a commonsense etiology. . . . Physicians take such a story, interrogate and expand it, all the while transmuting it into medical information.

Sooner or later they will return it to the patient as a diagnosis, an interpretative retelling that points toward the story's ending. In this way, much of the central business of caring for patients is transacted by means of narrative.

This position is an important turn in thinking about medical practice, as it opens the door for a serious consideration of other ways of knowing, other forms of knowledge that are important in caring for the patient. It should also be noted that in all of the alternative or competing views described previously, the patient's story is, in one way or another, moved to center stage and thus there is either an explicit or implicit move toward narrative conceptions of medical practice. In Chapter 2 we shall look carefully at this narrative turn, but for now, we finish this chapter with the thoughts of cognitive psychologist Jerome Bruner, and social psychologist Theodore Sarbin, about two ways of knowing our world, for they are an indirect critique of the prevailing way of knowing in biomedicine.

In 1985, Bruner (35) published "Narrative and Paradigmatic Modes of Thought" in the *Yearbook of the National Society for the Study of Education.*[*] In 1986, he expanded these arguments in the hallmark book *Actual Minds, Possible Worlds* (36). In the same year, Theodore Sarbin (37) edited a volume of essays directed at what many in social psychology were characterizing as an "epistemological crisis." In the cognitive psychology of Bruner and the social psychology of Sarbin and his colleagues we see a clear argument for using narrative as a root metaphor for the understanding of human behavior and a rejection of the hegemony of a positivist paradigm for the conduct of science. We find it instructive to quote Bruner's thesis on knowledge, as it is an insightful representation of the general position of social scientists of various persuasions. In his astute fashion, Bruner (35: 97) details the distinction between logico-scientific thinking (paradigmatic thinking) and narrative thinking:[†]

> There are two irreducible modes of cognitive functioning – or more simply, two modes of thought . . . each provides a way of ordering experience, of constructing reality, and the two (though amenable to complimentary use) are irreducible to one another. . . . Each of the ways of knowing . . . has operating principles of its own and its own criteria of well-formedness. But they differ radically in their procedures for establishing truth. One verifies by appeal to formal

---

[*] An earlier version of these ideas was given as an invited address to the American Psychological Association meeting in Toronto in 1984.

[†] Bruner recognizes that the distinction between two forms of knowledge has a long history and did not originate with him. In the late 1800s, the German philosopher Wilhelm Dilthey argued that what fundamentally distinguished the natural sciences from the human sciences was that the former aimed at developing causal explanations through the use of general laws, whereas the later aimed at understanding meaning from the person's point of view by grasping her subjective consciousness.

verification procedures and empirical proof. The other establishes *not* truth but truth-likeness or verisimilitude . . . the one seeks explications that are context free and universal, and the other seeks explications that are context sensitive and particular.

Bruner's argument, like that of Sarbin and other psychologists of the period, is a reaction to profound discontent about the imbalance in honoring these two modes of thought in the study of human behavior. After all, the *raison d'etre* among contributors to American social science was the belief that systematic inquiry into social circumstances of life would lead to information that could inform actions to benefit individual and collective action.

And so it is now time to consider a question that lurks under the surface of the argument in this chapter. What accounts for the tenacious hold by medicine and the social and behavioral sciences on the assumptions of a widely discredited seventeenth-century view of science?

We believe that factors at two different sociocultural levels account for this phenomenon. At a macro level, several scholars have argued that Western cultural traditions and the expressed value for monotheism have influenced the normal practice of biomedicine (1, 38–41). For example, Kleinman (1: 27) has speculated as follows:*

> The idea of a single god legitimates the idea of a single, underlying, universalizable truth, a unitary paradigm. Tolerance for alternative paradigms is weak or absent. . . . Alternatives may persist in the popular culture or at the professional fringe, but they are execrated as false beliefs by the profession as a whole, not unlike the accusation of heresy in the Western religious tradition. . . . At least this is the way biomedicine and the Western tradition look from the non-Western world, inasmuch as Chinese and Ayurvedic medical traditions tolerate alternative competing paradigms, seem less troubled by the uncertainty of human experience, and are more pluralistic in their theoretical orientations and therapeutic practices . . .

Kleinman suggests that the idea of monotheism unavoidably, unknowingly, and unreflectively supports a single-minded approach to disease within a biomedical model that seeks to uncover root causes in the service of diagnoses that are certain and precise.

From a cross-cultural perspective, thinking in terms of dualisms is more characteristic of Western cultures (e.g. male–female, mind–body, hard–soft, strength–weakness). In biomedicine, this dualistic way of framing the world leads to notions of "hard science" and "soft science", along with an associated value

---

* We take speculation to be a statement that cannot be falsified, but important in that it drives interest and study. It leads to new observations and then to useful knowledge.

system. Those areas of medicine that are perceived to be "hard" (procedural and technology-driven areas such as surgery) are valued more than the "soft" talk and cognitive-driven areas (such as psychiatry and primary care disciplines). The cultural and economic pressure within the profession is for the "soft" disciplines to become more procedure based and therefore more credible – more scientific.

At a micro level there are at least two factors that contribute to contemporary medicine's restricted view of what constitutes quality health care. First and foremost, too many physicians are unaware of current developments in the history and philosophy of science and in the work of the social sciences and humanities as these pertain to medicine. Furthermore, medical training at all levels remains too narrowly focused, so graduates have a very restricted view of the human condition. At best, an overwhelming majority of medical and nursing students, residents, nurses, and physicians have had only superficial exposure to the medical humanities and social sciences (14, 42–46).

Secondly, there is a pervasive misunderstanding among many practicing physicians and nurses of the limitations and boundaries of biomedicine. Too few practitioners have a nuanced appreciation of twenty-first-century models of scientific and narrative ways of knowing. Again, this condition is often the result of a lack of understanding about the ideas that are historically foundational to the profession. Aristotle spoke to three intellectual virtues, namely science or scientific knowledge (*episteme*), craft knowledge based on technical intelligence (*techne*), and ethics or practical moral knowledge – wisdom (*phronesis*). Over time, what has happened in medicine is that *episteme* has been assimilated into *techne*, resulting in scientism and a mistaken belief that technology constitutes science. *Phronesis* has been assimilated into *techne*, thus disregarding the relevance of hermeneutics to the human condition, and medicine values and legitimizes a caricatured version of science (*episteme*) over practical wisdom (*phronesis*).*

These macro and micro forces combine to provide a powerful culture of resistance to seriously considering alternative paradigms for the theory and clinical practice of medicine. So we come full circle and return to the clinical story that opens this chapter.

Why wasn't the physician "aware of this man's piano playing, and further-more of how important it was to him"? The dominant storyline is the patient's disease – his irreparable kidneys. The patient's body viewed as a machine with defective parts is the focus of his technologically driven medical care. Under these circumstances, the doctors involved in his treatment gather "objective" information by taking a physician-driven medical history, performing laboratory tests and intervening with surgery to "fix" the physical problem. By accepted standards of biomedical care, the patient has received "appropriate and good"

---

* The social scientist and philosopher, Bent Flyvbjerg (47), has argued convincingly for a similar situation in the social and behavioral sciences. These disciplines, too, have lost sight of their original purposes, resulting in an all too often uninformed dogmatic allegiance to *techne*, with a concomitant loss in practical wisdom (*phronesis*).

care. The physicians have acted in the best interests of the patient, given their biomedically driven framework. This is the medical story that is privileged. And given this framework, these "biases", rooted as they are in seventeenth- to nineteenth-century ideas of science and medical practice, the patient's illness story is silenced. The personhood of this patient doesn't matter to the repair of the damaged body part. Only when the medical student, who has not been fully socialized into the historically influenced form of medical practice followed by senior physicians, pursues the patient's sense of self, and honors the patient's illness story, are the physicians in a position to care for the person and not just the broken body part. What is important to the patient and is his source of suffering is the lack of full function of his hand from the surgical procedure, and the consequences of this impairment for his identity as a pianist. If the act of "complaining" – the patient's narrative of discontent and suffering – had been valued, attended to, witnessed, and honored, both patient and physician would have been humanized rather than dehumanized. Acting with narrative competence by turning seriously to the patient's illness narrative would have led the physicians in this case toward different treatment methods and different outcomes. Narrative knowledge and biomedical knowledge could have been balanced and integrated to enact a better outcome and a stronger affiliation between two human beings.

In the end, almost as a serendipitous event, the physician is transformed because of the power of the patient's narrative both to the patient and to what it means to be a doctor. And so the questions become the following. What is a narrative turn in health care and what does it mean for patient care? We shall explore these issues in the next chapter.

FURTHER ACTIVITIES

1 Readers who are interested in the history and philosophy of medicine are encouraged to read the following key texts:
   • Starr P. *The Social Transformation of American Medicine: the rise of a sovereign profession and the making of a vast industry.* New York: Basic Books; 1982.
   • Ludmerer K. *Time to Heal: American medical education from the turn of the century to the era of managed care.* New York: Oxford University Press; 1999.
   • Porter R. *The Greatest Benefit to Mankind: a medical history of humanity.* New York: Norton; 1997.
   • Dingwall HM. *A History of Scottish Medicine.* Edinburgh: University of Edinburgh Press; 2003.
2 In contrast to Descartes' notion of duality, consider the following poem by the Buddhist philosopher Thich Nhat Hanh (48). What does this philosophy of non-duality suggest about the relationship between patient and physician, and about the physician and herself?

Non-Duality

The bell tolls at four in the morning.
I stand by the window,
barefoot on the cool floor.
The garden is still dark.
I wait for the mountains and rivers to reclaim their shapes.
There is no light in the deepest hours of the night.
Yet, I know you are there
in the depth of the night,
the immeasurable world of the mind.
You, the known, have been there
ever since the knower has been.

The dawn will come soon,
and you will see
that you and the rosy horizon
are within my two eyes.
It is for me that the horizon is rosy
and the sky blue.
Looking at your image in the clear stream,
you answer the question by your presence.

Life is humming the song of the non-dual marvel.
I suddenly find myself smiling
in the presence of this immaculate night.
I know because I am here that you are there,
and your being has returned to show itself
in the wonder of tonight's smile.
In the quiet stream,
I swim gently.
The murmur of the water lulls my heart.
A wave serves as a pillow.
I look up and see
a white cloud against the blue sky,
the sound of autumn leaves,
the fragrance of hay –
each one a sign of eternity.
A bright star helps me find my way back to myself.

I know because you are there that I am here.
The stretching arm of cognition
in a lightning flash,
joining together a million eons of distance,
joining together birth and death,
joining together the known and the knower.

In the depth of the night,
as in the immeasurable realm of consciousness,
the garden of life and I
remain each other's objects.
The flower of being is singing the song of emptiness.

The night is still immaculate,
but sounds and images from you
have returned and fill the pure night.
I feel their presence.
By the window, with my bare feet on the cool floor,
I know I am here
for you to be.

Thich Nhat Hanh

REFERENCES

1 Kleinman A. *Writing at the Margin: discourse between anthropology and medicine.* Berkley, CA: University of California Press; 1995.

2 Lown B. *Bernard Lown: the lost art of healing;* www.humanmedia.org (accessed on 18 March 2008).

3 Starr P. *The Social Transformation of American Medicine: the rise of a sovereign profession and the making of a vast industry.* New York: Basic Books; 1982.

4 Ludmerer K. *Learning to Heal: the development of American medical education.* New York: Basic Books; 1985.

5 Ludmerer K. *Time to Heal: American medical education from the turn of the century to the era of managed care.* New York: Oxford University Press; 1999.

6 Porter R. *The Greatest Benefit to Mankind: a medical history of humanity.* New York: Norton; 1997.

7 Dingwall HM. *A History of Scottish Medicine.* Edinburgh: University of Edinburgh Press; 2003.

8 Brodsky A. *Benjamin Rush: patriot and physician.* New York: St Martin's Press; 2004.

9 Reiser SJ. *Medicine and the Reign of Technology.* Cambridge: Cambridge University Press; 1978.

10 Holmes OW. The Stethoscope Song, A professional ballad. In: Reynolds R, Stone J, editors. 3rd ed. *On Doctoring: stories, poems, essays.* New York: Simon & Schuster; 2001. pp. 25–6.

11 McWhinney IR. Why we need a new clinical method. In: Stewart M, Brown JB, Weston WW *et al.,* editors. *Patient-Centered Medicine: transforming the clinical method.* Thousand Oaks, CA: Sage; 1995. pp. 1–18.

12 McWhinney IR. The evolution of clinical method. In: Stewart M, Brown JB, Weston WW *et al.,* editors. *Patient-Centered Medicine: transforming the clinical method.* Thousand Oaks, CA: Sage; 2003. pp. 17–30.

13 Foss L, Rothenberg K. *The Second Medical Revolution: from biomedicine to infomedicine.*

Boston, MA: Shambala; 1987.

14 Odegaard CE. *Dear Doctor: a personal letter to a physician.* Menlo Park, CA: The Henry J Kaiser Family Foundation; 1986.

15 Anderson FHH. *Francis Bacon: his career and his thought.* Berkeley, CA: University of California Press; 1962.

16 Osherson S, AmaraSingham L. The machine metaphor in medicine. In: Mishler E, Mishler G, AmaraSingham L, editors. *Social Contexts of Health, Illness and Patient Care.* New York: Cambridge University Press; 1981. pp. 218–49.

17 Sullivan M. In what sense is contemporary medicine dualistic? *Cult Med Psychiatry.* 1986; **10**: 331–50.

18 Kuhn TS. *The Structure of Scientific Revolutions.* 2nd ed. Chicago, IL: University of Chicago Press; 1970.

19 Whitehead AN. *Science and the Modern World.* San Francisco, CA: Collins Fontana; 1975.

20 Toulmin S. *Cosmopolis: the hidden agenda of modernity.* Chicago, IL: University of Chicago Press; 1992.

21 Cassell E. The changing concept of the ideal physician. *Daedalus.* 1986; **115(2)**: 185–208.

22 Engel G. How much longer must medicine's science be bound by a seventeenth-century world view? In: White KL, editor. *The Task of Medicine: dialogue at Wickenburg.* Menlo Park, CA: The Henry J Kaiser Family Foundation; 1988. pp. 113–36.

23 Schwartz MA, Wiggins OP. Science, humanism, and the nature of medical practice: a phenomenological view. *Perspect Bio Med.* 1985; **28**: 331–61.

24 Pellegrino ED. Foreword. In: Mayock PP, editor. *Scott Buchanan: the doctrine of signatures: a defense of theory in medicine.* Urbana, IL: University of Illinois Press; 1991. pp. ix–xiii.

25 Powles J. On the limitations of modern medicine. In: *Science, Medicine and Man. Volume 1.* London: Pergamon Press; 1973. pp. 1–30.

26 Kleinman A, Eisenberg L, Good B. Culture, illness and care. *Ann Intern Med.* 1978; **88**: 251–8.

27 Kleinman A. *The Illness Narratives: suffering, healing and the human condition.* New York: Basic Books; 1988.

28 Engel G. The need for a new medical model: a challenge for biomedicine. *Science.* 1977; **196**: 129–36.

29 Engel G. From biomedical to biopsychosocial. I. Being scientific in the human domain. *Fam Syst Health.* 1996; **14**: 425–33.

30 Schwartz MA, Wiggins OP. Scientific and humanistic medicine: a theory of clinical methods. In: White K, editor. *The Task of Medicine.* Menlo Park, CA: Henry J Kaiser Family Foundation; 1988.

31 McWhinney IR. Foreword. In: Foss L. *The End of Modern Medicine: biomedical science under a microscope.* New York: State University of New York Press; 2002. pp. ix–xiii.

32 Charon R. *Narrative Medicine: honoring the stories of illness.* New York: Oxford University Press; 2006.

33 Brody H. *Stories of Sickness.* 2nd ed. New York: Oxford University Press; 2003.

34 Hunter KM. *Doctors' Stories: the narrative structure of medical knowledge.* Princeton, NJ: Princeton University Press; 1991.

35 Bruner J. Narrative and paradigmatic modes of thought. In: Eisner E, editor. *Learning and Teaching the Ways of Knowing. Eighty-Fourth Yearbook of the National Society for the Study of Education, Part II.* Chicago, IL: National Society for the Study of Education; 1985. pp. 97–115.

36 Bruner J. *Actual Minds, Possible Worlds.* Cambridge, MA: Harvard University Press; 1986.

37 Sarbin TR, editor. *Narrative Psychology: the storied nature of human conduct.* New York: Praeger; 1986.

38 Gordon DR. Tenacious assumptions in Western medicine. In: Lock M, Gordon D, editors. *Biomedicine Examined.* Boston, MA: Kluwer Academic Publishers; 1988. pp. 19–56.

39 Leslie C, Young A. *Paths to Asian Medical Knowledge.* Berkeley, CA: University of California Press; 1992.

40 Unschuld P. Traditional Chinese medicine: some historical and epistemological reflections. *Soc Sci Med.* 1987; **24:** 1023–9.

41 Connolly WE. *Political Theory and Modernity.* Ithaca, NY: Cornell University Press; 1993.

42 Snow CP. Human care. *JAMA.* 1973; **225:** 617–21.

43 White K. *The Task of Medicine.* Menlo Park, CA: Henry J Kaiser Family Foundation; 1988.

44 Engel JD, Jones DL. Medicine as humanities. In: Mujumdar SK, Rosenfeld LM, Nash DB, Audet AM, editors. *Medicine and Health Care into the Twenty-First Century.* Easton, PA: Pennsylvania Academy of Sciences; 1995. pp. 409–31.

45 Evans M. Reflections on the humanities in medical education. *Med Educ.* 2002; **36:** 508–13.

46 Association of American Medical Colleges. *Learning Objectives for Medical Student Education: guidelines for medical schools.* Washington, DC: Association of American Medical Colleges; 1998.

47 Flyvbjerg B. *Making Social Science Matter: why social inquiry fails and how it can succeed again.* New York: Cambridge University Press; 2001.

48 Nhat Hanh T. *Call Me By My True Names: the collected poems of Thich Nhat Hanh.* Berkeley, CA: Parallax Press; 1999.

CHAPTER 2

Transdisciplinary Narrative Turns and Narrative Health Care

> Story is no longer in the spotlight, but the lamp by which other things are seen.
>
> **Martin Kreiswirth (1: 62)**

- ● **THE NATURE OF NARRATIVE IN DISCIPLINE AND PROFESSION**
  - — Narrative Naturalists
  - — Narrative Constructivists
- ● **NARRATIVE IDENTITY**
  - — The Temporality of Experience
  - — The Temporality of Action
  - — The Temporality of Selfhood and Life
- ● **NARRATIVE AND HEALTH CARE**
  - — Sickness, Life Stories, and Narrative Identity
  - — Patient–Physician Encounters
  - — Barriers Between Patients and Physicians
  - — Narrative Features of Care and Caring
  - — Narrative Competence
  - — Narrative Contexts
- ● **CODA**

KEY IDEAS

- Stories are a universal way of giving meaning to experience.
- Self-identity and self-understanding develop through narrative. Our identity is constructed as a continual process through the stories we tell to ourselves and to others.
- Unity and uniqueness of the self is achieved through the coherence of a person's life story – narrative coherence. Sickness ushers in a lived sense of discontinuity, a disruption in the coherence of a person's life narrative and identity.
- Four barriers divide physicians from their patients and make it difficult for physicians to work with patients to "repair" their illness stories. These barriers are understanding of mortality, contexts of illness, beliefs about disease causality, and emotions of shame, blame, and fear.
- Five features of narrative serve to reduce the distance between physicians and patients. These are temporality, singularity, causality, inter-subjectivity, and ethicality.

THE NATURE OF NARRATIVE IN DISCIPLINE AND PROFESSION

In the previous chapter we discussed various models of medicine that have been offered as alternatives to the dominant biomedical model. Common to all of these alternatives is the importance of narrative as a way of knowing about the patient and the physician as people as well as role incumbents. The biomedical model represents an overarching or grand narrative, and the alternative models represent small or local narratives that work in opposition to the hegemony of the grand narrative.* Medicine's turn to incorporate local narratives is a subset of a general turn toward taking narrative as a valued way of knowing and understanding for a wide range of social and behavioral phenomena. In this chapter, we examine narrative and how it has influenced a wide array of humanities and social science disciplines and several helping professions, medicine in particular, in the USA. Following this, we argue that narrative and self-identity are intimately linked, and thus stories represent the core of our identities. Relating the philosophical aspects of narrative to health care, we argue that illness experiences serve to disrupt these stories, and thus our identities. We conclude this chapter with a discussion of barriers that separate physicians from patients in the work of treating the patient's illness story, as well as what may be done to overcome these divides and restore care and caring to the relationship.

Beginning around the early 1980s, narrative seriously entered the theory and practice of multiple disciplines, including science and technology (2),

---

* This distinction is noted by Kreiswirth (1) and based on terminology used by Jean-Francois Lyotard. We simply reiterate it here. According to Kreiswirth (1: 71), '. . . grand narratives exert totalizing and, in some instances, totalitarian control, through the universalization of a particular plot, which restrictively positions its agents, narrators, and listeners.'

philosophy (3–9), history (10–12), psychology (13–18), the human sciences (19, 20), sociolinguistics (21–24), sociology (25–29), and anthropology (30). Several professions have incorporated the ideas of narrative into their academic and professional practice, including law (14, 31, 32), career counseling (33–36), education (37–39), occupational therapy (40), nursing (41–45), health policy (46), and medicine (47–52). Writing about these movements, Kreiswirth (1: 63) notes:

> . . . the recent obsession with narrative forms of interpretation and understanding as a response to . . . our current climate of anti-foundationalism, poststructuralism, and/or postmodernism – a response, that is, to the breakdown of transcendental truth-claims, to various overturnings or assaults on formerly hegemonic logico-deductive and patriarchal models of reason and knowledge.

This dramatic interest in narrative may be seen as a counter-revolution to the dominant paradigm within the respective disciplines and professions inventoried above. As Kreiswirth (19) has noted, the sociocultural context of the disciplines changed and allowed the theory and practice of narrative to move from the distant periphery toward the center of professional work and thought.

However, we don't want to leave the reader with the impression that narrative burst *de novo* on to the disciplinary scene. Certainly stories existed in these contexts, but they did so only as ornament – as a supplement to the serious business of the discipline. An interesting anecdote related to us recently by a colleague reminded us that the *British Medical Journal (BMJ)* has published narratives for years. They typically appeared at the end of each issue, and there were no page numbers assigned to them (i.e. they were of no scientific value and could not be referenced in the traditional way).

Although the sense of narrative or story varies across as well as within these professions and disciplines, there are some common features and issues that draw them together for a narrative turn in theory and practice. What is agreed upon is that stories or narratives are a universally human way of giving meaning to experience. They are a primary way in which we understand ourselves and the world we inhabit, and they are a primary means of influencing others. Once heard, a story initiates for the listener a search for possible meanings. Stories are dynamic, and evolve as people tell them and as they are listened to (19, 53).

Of course, as with most change in ideas and practice, the place of narrative within the intellectual and practical work of many disciplines and professions has come in overlapping phases and with other intellectual/cultural turns.* Kreiswirth (19: 296) writes:

---

* Several other "turns" within and across disciplines preceded the narrative turn. First there was a linguistic turn, followed by rhetorical and then interpretive turns. These shifts in theory and practice have been chronicled by several authors (54–57).

Since about 1980, the study of narrative has gradually moved away from what were then dominant semiotic or narratological perspectives, focused primarily on literary texts – the narrative turn's first phase – and then on to examinations of narrative as much in nontextual as in textual forms, as it related not only to cultural products but also to communication theory, pedagogy, sociology, cognition, therapy, memory, jurisprudence, politics, language acquisition, and artificial intelligence. . . . To oversimplify a bit, one might say that speculation about narrative was previously functional, formal, generic, or hermeneutic – we wanted to know what might make up its parts, how it might work, how it might be differentiated from other discursive forms, what it might mean . . . today we are examining narrative's ontology, politics, epistemology, ideology, cognitive status, and disciplinarity . . .

Interest in and work on these current issues by many theoreticians are driven in part by a concern that people's stories are so ubiquitous, so ordinary in everyday life, that their status as a paradigm for trustworthy knowledge and action is problematic. Is the patient story that began Chapter 1 a story with a claim for critical knowledge (storied knowledge) or is it merely a story, an ornament in a more trustworthy biomedical account? Those engaged in narrative work in the human sciences, medicine being one of the latter, argue that people's stories represent reality (ontological status) and portray trustworthy knowledge (epistemological status).* Kreiswirth (19) describes two perspectives on the ontologic and epistemic status of narrative – those of narrative naturalists and narrative constructivists. The differences in their positions are theoretically informative, so we shall now briefly look at each position.

Narrative Naturalists

The work of psychologist Jerome Bruner (13) is a good example of the naturalist position. He posits two fundamental modes of thought – logico-scientific (paradigmatic) and narrative. Each provides a different way of thinking about experience or reality. As Kreiswirth (19: 305) notes:

> The narrated . . . is a way of thinking whose form may get represented discursively as narrative; but the narration can claim a certain epistemic status because mind itself works through a process of narrative patterning . . . story does not discursively impose order on an inchoate flow of mental materials . . . rather it displays the narrative means by which the mind functions . . . story is not merely invented, but develops naturally as part of our conceptual and cognitive machinery . . .

---

* We recognize that truth in stories can only be partial. Stories, no matter how carefully rendered, can never fully portray the situation that they represent, since they are told from the narrator's point of view with details that are selectively chosen and remembered. However, stories' ontological and epistemological status is pragmatically sufficient to transact meaningful and important matters.

According to this theoretical view, language serves narrative by providing the cognitive basis for it (58). Interestingly, recent work in the neurosciences may support this position. Here, in three extended passages from his hallmark work, we provide the argument made by Laurence Foss (59: 141–3), the eminent philosopher of science referenced in Chapter 1.

> We have presented the infomedical case that the mid-brain has receptors for ideas, like those embedded in a novel, and these ideas can be transduced via well-defined channels to selectively affect cellular behavior. Upon receipt of a certain cognitive-affective message [a story], the pituitary might send hormones to glands such as the adrenal cortex and the ovaries and testes. These in turn can "secrete steroid hormones that penetrate into cells and direct the genes to synthesize proteins. These proteins then function as structural elements, enzymes, or vesicles that activate other cellular functions." (60: 130) (insertion and emphasis added)
>
> In this science, pathogenesis has three, not two, distinct etiological constraints. There are external physical environmental constraints, thus viruses and blistering factory chemicals. Call these *germs*. There are also internal biophysical, somatic constraints, like aberrant chemical reactions and defective nucleic acid sequences. Call these *genes*. Finally, there are internal psychobiophysical, extrasomatic constraints like concepts, emotions and neuroses. These are symbols or "*memes*", self-replicating, psychosocial information units. The need for including this third category originates with the observation that at a certain organizational level, systems evolve such that semantic behavior is superordinate to and, under certain conditions, can override or supplement laws governing somatic, that is autonomic, biological behavior. The human placebo response exemplifies this superordination.
>
> Key to the infomedical application of the meme concept . . . is the degree to which we as humans, rather than simply victims of our memes and genes, can exercise some individual and collective dominion over our memes – and through them our genes . . . consider the mundane meme, "My glass is half-full." Along with its counterpart, "My glass is half-empty", for infomedicalists, each is capable of influencing our biology, one for good (health), the other for ill (dis-ease). And as intentional, free-willing creatures, we have some choice over which meme we appropriate for our own in any given circumstance. One use of cognitive–behavioral therapies – guided imagery, biofeedback, and hypnotherapy are examples – is to enhance the exercise of these meme choices and so to influence our health. . . . Anorexics can lose weight even on regimens where extra calories are *consumed well beyond the minimum required to sustain basal metabolism.* And the conjectured reason is that the mid-brain, through the messages it sends (transduced via

messenger molecules), can actually alter the metabolism in such a way that the calories are burned up instead of stored as fat. An image or belief [**a story**], a "memetic" vector, interacts with metabolism, the offspring of genetic instructions. (insertion and emphasis added)

This expanded diagnostic category, the meme, is certainly interesting speculation, with some substantiation in recent neuroscience work (61, 62). In a general sense, this work supports the arguments of Jerome Bruner (13) and Mark Turner (58), which place narrative in the fundamental cognitive constitution of the individual and the species. This development could provide compelling warrant for privileging a patient's story in her care and treatment.*

Narrative Constructivists

In contrast to narrative naturalists, social or narrative constructivists argue that stories are formed, or constructed, from an interaction of lived experience through time and meaning. Thus temporality figures prominently in an essentially phenomenological or existential framework. Constructivists are skeptical of the naturalists' position that makes narrative a fundamental mental operation.

Paul Ricoeur, one of the leading French philosophers of the twentieth century, has focused his work on bridging phenomenology and language analysis. His body of work provides a phenomenological/hermeneutic basis for narrative in the human sciences. For Ricouer (6: 3), time and narrative are intimately related:

> . . . what is ultimately at stake in the case of the structural identity of the narrative function, as well as in that of the truth claim of every narrative work, is the temporal character of human experience. The world unfolded by every narrative work is always a temporal world . . . time becomes human time to the extent that it is organized after the manner of a narrative; narrative, in turn, is meaningful to the extent that it portrays the features of temporal experience.

And how does narrative portray the features of temporal experience? Ricoeur's answer is to embrace and differentiate Aristotle's idea of mimesis (63). By mimesis, Aristotle meant an imaginative re-description of an action accomplished in such a way as to represent essential patterns and meanings that were latent. Kearney (64: 132) writes:

> Mimesis is "invention" in the original sense of that term: *invenire* means both to discover *and* to create, that is, to disclose what is already there

---

* This work supports a general mind–body connection, and is consistent with work in fields such as psychoneuroimmunology.

in the light of what is not yet (but is potentially). It is the power, in short, to re-create actual worlds as possible worlds.

Consequently, mimesis is linked intimately to Aristotle's notion of mythos or plot – a weaving together of past, present, and future. Ricoeur (6) differentiates Aristotle's notion of mimesis by describing what he refers to as *threefold mimesis* (*mimesis₁*, *mimesis₂*, *mimesis₃*). Kearney (64: 133) discusses these three stages:

> This brings me . . . to what Ricoeur calls the circle of triple *mimesis*: (1) the *prefiguring* of our life-world as it seeks to be told; (2) the *configuring* of the text in the act of telling; and (3) the *refiguring* of our existence as we return from narrative text to action. This referral of narrative back to the life of the author and forward to the life of the reader . . . is why we insist that the act of *mimesis* involves a circular movement from action to text and back again – passing from prefigured experience through narrative recounting back to a refigured life-world.

Charon (48: 138), in discussing *threefold mimesis*, links the three stages to what she refers to as three movements in narrative medicine (attention, representation, and affiliation), and notes:

> Not unlike what I have been calling *attention*, mimesis₁ brings the human agent freshly and openly in front of whatever is to be beheld so as to free from it its meaning. . . . If Ricoeur's mimesis₁ corresponds to . . . "attention", mimesis₂ corresponds to "representation." . . . Looking ahead to . . . affiliation, mimesis₃ gives us terms with which to establish the fact that actual clinical actions – of therapeutic engagement and building of collegial community – are the inevitable and powerful dividends of achieving attention and representation.

For narrative temporalists such as Ricoeur, the narrative act is not related to the fundamental workings of cognition. It is, in their view, the particular aspects of cognition that deal with thinking in and through time that provide humans with a storied existence. As noted by Kreisworth (19), Charon (48), Ricoeur (65), and Taylor (66), among others, this position brings with it a particular interest in the construction and reconstruction of self-identity, biography, and autobiography. For these theorists, story portrays the sense we have of ourselves and others as essentially moral agents, as people expressing agency through time – past, present, and future. On this point, the philosopher and political scientist, Charles Taylor (66: 47), suggests that:

> . . . to make minimal sense of our lives . . . to have an identity, we need an orientation to the good . . . this sense of good has to be woven into my understanding of my life as an unfolding story. But this is to state

> another basic condition of making sense of ourselves, that we grasp
> our lives in a *narrative*... making sense of one's life as a story is... not
> an optional extra; that our lives exist also in this space of questions,
> which only a coherent narrative can answer. In order to have a sense
> of who we are, we have a notion of how we have become, and of where
> we are going ...

This idea of self-identity and self-understanding through the temporality of narrative is particularly important in an overwhelming majority of perspectives on narrative. However, before turning to a deeper exploration of this idea, we should note one other view of narrative construction.

Some theorists, following one of the variations of critical social theory, choose to highlight the cultural politics of self-identity and self-understanding through narrative. For example, the physician and critical sociologist, Howard Waitzkin (67), argues that social, political, and economic factors as well as cultural institutions influence the way that personal narratives are constructed and transmitted. From this perspective, stories function as both constraining and liberating mechanisms with regard to how people construct and enact the moral space which they inhabit.* The point here is that some theorists remind us that narratives often have their origin in factors external to the individual, and consequently need to be queried for hidden values and agendas that serve to distort meaning and representation.

Given the various perspectives on the nature of narrative, we believe that while the philosophical preferences between naturalists and constructivists are theoretically instructive and provide important speculation for research, the differences at the present time seem to matter less at the level of clinical practice. Although we tend to be critical social constructivists, our position is a critical pragmatic one that frames the origin of personal narratives in the dynamic of a cognitively based subjective experience lived through time and culture. Given this position, the stage is set for a discussion of connections among the concepts of self-identity and narrative. Here our tendency is to follow the ideas most closely associated with varieties of phenomenology and existentialism.

NARRATIVE IDENTITY†

Along with the turn to narrative comes a position, taken by several theorists from different disciplinary viewpoints (literary theory, sociology, and philosophy),

---

* The sociopolitical narrative perspective, when taken to extremes, becomes essentially an anti-narrative position. Narrative in this extreme version is not to be trusted. It has become strongly influenced by ideology, framed by grand narratives that serve to silence local and particularistic narratives. For more information about sociopolitical narratives, see Rosenwald and Ochberg (68) and Skultans (69).

† The term "narrative identity" was originated by Shlomith Rimmon-Kenan (70), and we are indebted to her for developing the idea.

that self-identity and narrative are intimately linked and that stories are at the core of our identities (70–75).* These distinct disciplinary orientations to narrative each have different implications for the link between narrative and self. For present purposes, we choose to focus on commonalities across various disciplines/viewpoints. It is important to note here that we are primarily interested in non-fictional narratives. Hence the extensive corpus of theoretical work concerned with fictional narrative will be brought into play when it helps us to understand our primary focus. Although from time to time we may acknowledge the debates within and across disciplines, we will not spend time rehearsing them, since we believe that often they have little relevance for those practicing narratively in health care. Our preferred viewpoint is based on intellectual work in the social sciences. However, we recognize, value, and utilize, in pragmatic ways, ideas associated with the theoretical positions of other disciplines. In point of fact, most work today is interdisciplinary – a sign of our postmodern times. That said, we begin with an examination of work that connects the ideas of narrative and self-identity.

Sarbin (18: 3, 9), in writing about narrative as a root metaphor for psychology, has argued that:

> A story is a symbolized account of actions of human beings that has a temporal dimension. The story has a beginning, middle and an ending. ... The story is held together by recognizable patterns of events called plots. Central to the plot structure are human predicaments and attempted solutions ...
>
> The narrative is a way of organizing episodes, actions, and accounts of actions; it is an achievement that brings together mundane facts and fantastic creations; time and space are incorporated. The narrative allows for the inclusion of actors' reasons for their acts, as well as the causes of happening.

Sarbin proposes a *narratory principle* as an organizer for human action and life. People *think, perceive, imagine, and make moral choices* within the structure of stories (18). The narrative psychology of Sarbin and other constructivists (14, 15, 20) attributes a central role to language, specifically stories, in the process of making oneself. Following these theorists, our contention is that we lead our lives through stories and that our identity is constructed as a continual process through the stories which we tell ourselves and about ourselves to others.

The narrative psychosocial viewpoint of human life draws heavily on phenomenological and existential approaches to reality. As noted above, such approaches have been particularly sensitive to the ways in which human beings routinely orient to time and place – we are historical beings. As Carr (10: 4)

---

* There is certainly a counter position which holds that stories of self do not constitute self, but rather deflect what is true self (*see*, for example, 76).

so beautifully puts it, ". . . we are in history as we are in the world: it serves as the horizon and background for our everyday experience." Carr's position is that human experience of everyday life has a narrative structure – a temporal configuration of events (a beginning, middle, and end), a narrator, and an audience.* Drawing from ideas of temporality framed by the phenomenology and existentialism of Husserl, Heidegger, Merleau-Ponty, and Dilthey, Carr explores the form of narrative embodied in the experience, action, and life of the individual. His analysis of three levels of human experience – the temporality of passive experience, the temporality of action, and the temporality of selfhood and life – is pertinent to our project.

The Temporality of Experience

In theorizing about the temporal features of human experience, Carr appropriates Husserl's theory of consciousness of ongoing events. According to Husserl, when we encounter events, even at the most passive level, they are infused with anticipation of the future (protention) and our memory of things past (retention). Carr (10: 23) notes: 'Taking the past and future horizons together, then, one may speak of the temporal as a "field of occurrence", in which the present stands out from its surroundings, and of our consciousness as a kind of gaze which "takes in" or spans the field in which the focal object stands out.' Thus events make up the temporal configurations that are the substance of our daily experience. He continues (10: 24): 'Even though as temporal they unfold bit by bit, we experience them as configurations thanks to our protentional and retentional "gaze" which spans future and past.' Thus our conscious experience of an event is inextricably intertwined with a temporal configuration of past–present–future that mutually determine each other as parts of a whole.

The Temporality of Action

Carr (10: 31) explores his thesis by observing that the greater part of our everyday lives is active rather than passive experience, stating that ". . . if our passive experience is characterized by a complex temporal structure, our active experience is all the more so. The key to this structure is the purposive or means-end character of action . . ." Carr notes that when we are involved in an action, the focus of our concern is in the future, not in the present. He notes (10: 39) that ". . . the future is salient while the present and the past constitute its background. This is one way . . . of rendering account of the difference between activity and passivity. Activity is future-centered . . . and is not simply *attention* but *intention* that is focused there . . ." Carr maintains that the means-end structure with its characteristic past–present–future configuration displays the same temporal, beginning–middle–end structure as narrative. The point is that present experience is only meaningful when framed in terms of a complex set of relational memories from the past and situational projections of and for the

---

* We are indebted to Crossley (15) for bringing to our attention the work of Carr.

future. Certainly his case is that the structure of passive and active experience is temporal and the key to this structure is its narrative character. Narrative structure is thus not something that is laid over experience to explain it, but rather it is in the nature of experience itself.

After considering the narrative structure of short-term elementary experiences, Carr turns his attention to the narrative structure of longer-term and larger-scale sequences of experiences, actions, and human events. On this issue, he states (10: 52–3):

> In our experience, events foreshadow, augment, and repeat other events so that the complex events they make up . . . are criss-crossed with lines of resemblance (to quote Hume), contiguity, and causality. . . . In the case of actions, again the structural features are carried over to a large scale. Actions which have their own means-end structure become means toward the performance of other actions . . .

This brings Carr to the related issue of how these larger scales, multiple experiences and actions are dealt with in a person's experience. His response is to hearken to the work of Schutz and invoke the idea of a reflexive or reflective grasp (10: 55):

> If the structure of complex experiences and actions can be considered a replica at a larger scale of the part-whole, beginning-middle-end structure of the simple phenomenon, it nevertheless requires a different subjective role on the part of the experiencer or agent. The subject is no longer immersed in the larger–scale phenomenon through a retentive-protentive awareness . . . when the larger-scale activity spans a multiplicity of actions or experiences, these must be held together by a grasp which attends not only to the object, or objective, but also to the disparate and temporally discrete parts of my experience or activity that render the object present or constitute my engagement in the action.

A key phrase in Carr's argument is *disparate and temporally discrete parts.* This signals the situation where there are interruptions in events. Here, as Carr points out, we are in a transition from retention and protention to recollection and expectation and perhaps deliberation and planning. He (10: 56) reminds us that "The recollection, expectation and deliberation . . . are practical concerns whose purpose is to organize or recognize these elements into a unified whole. Thus, the elements are taken together and considered in their interrelation. It is the whole as an interrelation of parts which becomes thematic." So, when my physician and I (*JDE*) discuss the results of a recent endoscopy of my esophagus and the appearance of precancerous cells identified on biopsy, the sense of where I stand in the long-term progression of my disease needs to be restored by an act of recollection and reflection, so that planning around my illness can proceed in such a way as to maintain continuity of my life story. Recollections and reflections are criss-crossed by my memories of a dear friend who suffered with and died of esophageal cancer. Notice that there is a network of social and cultural reciprocity involved in constructing a human life and illness as narrative.

The Temporality of Selfhood and Life

Carr then turns to the third level of human experience – that of selfhood and life. Here he theorizes that the conception of narrative structure of experience is also the organizing principle of the self who experiences and acts (10). The discussion of larger-scale sequences of experiences and actions finds its place at the level of life stories. A life story requires a reflective temporal grasp which takes all the separate stories together and establishes the connections among them.

Some authors, such as literary theorist Paul John Eakin (74: 101), have argued that this occurs through the process of autobiography which ". . . is properly understood as an integral part of a lifelong process of identity formation in which acts of self-narration play a major part." Here, Eakin separates lived first-person autobiography from literary autobiography. Literary autobiographies are biographical reflections being conducted in the present with a view to portraying the past. Lived biography is more often concerned with the past in order to make it coherent with or comprehensible in terms of a present and a future where the biographical past figures as a horizon in our actions. On this point, Carr (10: 75–6) states:

> . . . a multiplicity of activities and projects, spread out over time and even existing simultaneously in the present, calls for an active reflection that attempts to put the whole together. The most striking occasions for such reflections are those radical conversions . . . in which a new view of life, of oneself, and of one's future prospects requires a break with and reinterpretation of one's past . . . we are composing and constantly revising our autobiographies as we go along.

He claims (10: 61–2):

> To be an agent or subject of experience is to make the constant attempt to surmount time in exactly the way the story-teller does. It is the attempt to dominate the flow of events by gathering them together in the forward-backward grasp of the narrative act . . . narration constitutes something, creates meaning rather than just reflecting or imitating something that exists independently of it. But narration, intertwined as it is with action, does this in the course of life itself, not merely after the fact . . .

For Eakin (74: 101), similarly, the connection between narrative and self is profound: "Narrative and identity are performed simultaneously . . . in a single act of self-narration; the self in question is a self defined by and transacted in narrative process . . . narrative here is not merely *about* the self but rather in some profound way a constituent part *of* self . . ." Oliver Sacks (77: 110) offers a stronger version of this position: "It might be said that each of us constructs and lives a 'narrative', and that this narrative *is* us, our identities."

Thus we see that there is significant agreement across a wide variety of scholars that narration is an extension of a primary feature of reality, i.e. temporality. Furthermore, unity and uniqueness of the self are achieved through the coherence of a person's life story. Narrative coherence is the norm or rule, and Carr (10) shows this to be so in two ways. First, for most of us, for most of the time, things do hang together. And secondly, narrative coherence is the standard against which to judge narrative disarray. When things fall apart, when our plans fall apart, it is by reference to storied projections of life and self.

Charlotte Linde (23), an ethnographer–linguist, has conducted one of the few empirical studies of narrative and coherence. Her findings support the philosophical arguments of Carr and others. In a small case study of oral life story, concerning 13 white middle-class Americans and their choice of a profession, Linde focused on the social practice of creating, exchanging, and negotiating coherent life stories. She found that coherence is both a social demand and an internal psychological demand that involves work at three linguistic levels – narrative, coherence principles, and coherence systems. At the most basic level, the person creates a story that is coherent in a temporal sense so that the events are perceived as orderly over time. The coherence principles used in structuring a life story are causality and continuity. And at the highest level, a life story must adhere to social systems of assumptions about the world that make events coherent. Linde (23: 222) suggests that "The most pervasive and invisible coherence system is common sense – the set of beliefs and relations between beliefs that speakers may assume are known and shared by all competent members of the culture." It is precisely a sustained disruption in a coherent narrative identity with respect to a person's health status that initiates for most individuals an encounter with a health care provider. It is to this connection between narrative and medicine that we turn next.

NARRATIVE AND HEALTH CARE

As we have argued above, within many disciplines there has been a dramatically increased recognition of the importance and relevance of ideas about narrative for at least the last 30 years. This narrative turn, as we have seen, is connected to discussions of postmodernism. At the risk of oversimplifying, postmodernism is generally taken to be the intellectual period that challenges the objectivity of science and medicine, and argues that knowledge is primarily and importantly framed by culture, history, and language. Epistemology and ontology for many postmodernists are essentially narrative in character.

Health care, particularly medicine, has been slower to explore narrative views than other disciplines and professions. Until recently, except for departments and/or programs of medical sociology, anthropology, and humanities, medicine has not seriously incorporated ideas of narrative medicine. That condition has changed radically in the last few years, so much so that one can speak of a *narrative medicine movement*. Like most social–intellectual movements, the narrative movement is responsive to broader currents within medicine and culture at large. Movements such as feminism, consumerism, patient rights, and managed health care have set the stage for receptiveness within health care to the idea that life *is* a story. When health care practitioners interact with patients, they jointly are writing new chapters or revising existing chapters in their stories – both the patients' and their own stories. In turn, this process connects with another recent movement within medicine – *relationship-centered care*. This form of patient–physician relationship will be the focus of the next chapter. For now, we shall focus on the place of narrative in health care.

Beginning in the mid-1980s, a series of landmark books connecting narrative and the practice of health care was published, drawing explicitly and implicitly on the theoretical work being conducted on narrative identity. Here is a sampling of those works. In 1987, the first medical textbook with the term "stories" in the title appeared – *Stories of Sickness* by the family physician and philosopher Howard Brody (78). *The Illness Narratives: Suffering, Healing, and the Human Condition*, by the physician and anthropologist Arthur Kleinman (50), appeared the following year.* These two books by physicians mark an early *narrative turn* in health care. They are important works, as they gave voice and cultural legitimacy to the critical importance of the patient's story, and drew attention to the efficacy of subjective knowledge in the diagnosis and treatment of patients.

Kathryn Montgomery Hunter's *Doctor Stories: the Narrative Structure of Medical Knowledge* (79) appeared in 1991. In 1995, the medical sociologist and cancer survivor, Arthur Frank, published an influential volume entitled *The Wounded Storyteller: Body, Illness, and Ethics* (25). Anne Hudson Jones, a literary scholar, began a literature and medicine series in *The Lancet* in 1996. Hilde Lidemann Nelson, philosopher and ethicist, edited a collection entitled *Stories and Their Limits: Narrative Approaches to Bioethics* (80), published in 1997. *Narrative-Based Medicine: Dialogue and Discourse in Clinical Practice*, an edited volume by two British general practitioners, Trisha Greenhalgh and Brian Hurwitz (49), was published in 1998. In the same year, Cheryl Mattingly, anthropologist and occupational therapist, published *Healing Dramas and Clinical Plots: the Narrative Structure of Experience* (81). Following this, *Narrative-Based Primary Care*, authored by another British general practitioner, John Launer, (51) appeared in 2002. In 2006, Rita Charon, an internist and literary scholar at Columbia College of

---

* This work is an extended statement of ideas published 10 years earlier by Kleinman and his colleagues, Eisenberg and Good (*see* Chapter 1, reference 26).

Physicians and Surgeons, published *Narrative Medicine: Honoring the Stories of Illness* (48), and Trisha Greenhalgh published *What Seems to be the Trouble? Stories in Illness and Healthcare* (52).

To be sure, other works (including numerous journal articles) elucidating the place of narrative and stories in health care have been published. For example, listening to the patient's story – not only the clinical story of signs, symptoms, and onset of illness, but the patient's life story – was documented as part of the nursing role as far back as the days of Florence Nightingale. In 1859, Nightingale's *Notes on Nursing: What It Is, and What It Is Not* was first published. It established the practice of using patient narratives to persuade those in authority that reforms were needed in nursing training. Narrative as a term utilized to describe a path to knowledge in nursing care was first introduced in the *Cumulated Index of Nursing and Allied Health Literature* in 1997. Darbyshire (42, 43), Younger (44), and Sakalys (45) have produced important works that indicate the connection between nursing and narrative.

Today, we have a robust body of work connecting narrative theory and practice with medical theory and practice. Taken together, what is particularly interesting about these works is that they portray narrative health care as both a philosophy of care and a set of skills. Of course, represented in this body of work are different points of emphasis along with differences in details regarding what constitute important features of narrative and narrative care. The ideas of narrative health care are, after all, influenced by the intellectual traditions of those constructing the field. With diversity in philosophy, method, and practice, what is evolving is considerable commonality with regard to what narrative health care is, how it should be practiced, and how to educate professionals in the required skills. Charon's comments (82: 27–8) regarding narrative ethics, a core component of narrative medicine, apply just as well to all of narrative health care.

> What characterizes these approaches as "narrative" is that they take as given that each sick person enters sickness singularly, that each signifies differently, and that each death connotes the end of its life particularly. It is the ethos of narrative ethics that one must tell of what one undergoes in order to understand it and that, as a consequence, the health professionals who accompany one through illness have a responsibility to hear one out. Among the tenets of narrative ethics are the requirements to hear all sides, to contextualize all events, to honor all voices, and to bear witness to all who suffer. Training for such practice, it follows, is textual and interior – developing the skills of close reading, reflective discernment, self-knowledge, and absorptive and interpretive listening.

With this said, we turn first and primarily to describing the commonalities of narrative medicine as philosophy and as skills. The work of three physicians

– Charon, Greenhalgh, and Brody – seems to us to be the most comprehensive in describing narrative theory and practice as it relates to medicine as a field. We take our lead from them in portraying the general features of narrative health care in the related fields of medicine, nursing, and allied health. We acknowledge that each specific health care profession enacts narrative within the particular requirements of its professional context.

The collective work of these physicians can be mapped as follows:

> Narrative health care stakes out a fundamental position on the relationship among *sickness, life stories, and personal identity*. With this ontology in place, narrative health care supports particular enactments of *patient–physician encounters* and overcomes *barriers between patients and practitioners* through emphasizing *narrative features of care/caring* and by encouraging the development and enactment of *narrative competence* in a *variety of health care contexts*.

Each of the italicized terms represents a cluster of the key ideas from their work. Here we provide an overview of each set of terms. In Chapters 4, 5, and 6, we shall cover these ideas in greater detail. Readers who are unfamiliar with the works of Charon, Greenhalgh, and Brody are encouraged to examine those listed in the "Further Activities" section at the end of this chapter.

Sickness, Life Stories, and Narrative Identity

Brody, who is professionally trained in both medicine and philosophy, is concerned with a philosophical analysis of several concepts that are central to health care and that then set the place for narratives in clinical care. In Brody's analytic scheme (47: 44) there are five interrelated aspects of sickness:

1 To be sick is to have something wrong with oneself in a way regarded as abnormal when compared with a suitably chosen reference class.
2 To be sick is to experience both an unpleasant sense of disruption of body and self, and a threat to one's integrated personhood.
3 To be sick is to have the sort of thing that medicine, as an evolving craft, has customarily treated.
4 To be sick is to undergo an alteration of one's social roles and relationships in ways that will be influenced by cultural belief systems.
5 To be sick is to participate in a disruption of an integrated hierarchy of natural systems, including one's biological subsystems, oneself as a discrete psychological entity, and the social and cultural systems of which one is a member.

Sickness is conceptualized as a complex relationship among physical, socio-cultural, and existential dimensions. How are stories related to this analysis of sickness?

For narrativists such as Brody, the link is through personal identity. Because of Brody's training as a philosopher, he is well acquainted with the importance of this idea in twentieth-century Anglo-American philosophy, as well as the various arguments that constitute its treatment. Brody (47), rehearsing the work of Alasdair McIntyre (4), aligns his thinking with a narrative form of life and, consequently, with the narrative identity position described in the previous section. The connection between narrative identity and sickness comes when the patient's life story is interrupted by serious illness. As noted earlier in the work of Carr (10) and Linde (23), there is a social–psychological drive toward coherence in life story as a means of keeping the person's identity intact. Sickness brings with it a lived sense of discontinuity, a disruption in coherence of the person's life narrative and identity. On this issue, Rimmon-Kenan (70: 12–13) states:

> Continuity . . . is one form of coherence and the one that is specifically related to narrative, since it operates in time, time being a basic constituent of narrative. Continuity is a chronological linkage between three temporal dimensions; past, present, and future. It is this linkage, characteristic of both stories and "narrative identity", that is destabilized by illness . . . most illness narratives . . . tend . . . to retell, restructure past memories and future expectations in a way that would cohere with the present, bridging the gap by creating a new kind of continuity, or a continuity governed by different emphases.

Consistent with the work of Linde that was noted previously (23), Rimmon-Kenan (70: 14) goes on to say: "The pull toward coherence, continuity, transformation . . . is also affected by socially and culturally constructed expectations." And medical sociologist Mike Bury (83: 264) states: ". . . illness constitutes a major instance of 'biographical disruption' in which the relations between body, mind and everyday life are threatened."

Given this philosophical and empirical connection between narrative identity and illness, we maintain that each medical encounter ought to attend seriously to the patient's story. With this said, we need to continue focusing our attention on the particulars of forms of health care delivery.

Patient–Physician Encounters

In Chapters 3 and 4, we shall consider various types of patient–physician relationships. Here, we want to provide a sense of the connection between narrative and current models of medical care. Suffice it to say that recently there has been much discussion of and advocacy for models of care that have been variously conceived of as "patient-centered care", "sustained partnerships", "participatory decision making", and "relationship-centered care" (84, 85). With regard to these models, Brody (47: 66) writes:

> Despite differences in details, these models share important features that bring the patient's story front and center. They advocate a physician who takes a personal interest in the patient as a human being with whom she will relate over time. The physician is expected to view the patient as possessing an important base of expertise, without which the medical encounter cannot proceed. . . . The "storied" relationship between physician and patient is not being advocated merely because it is more compassionate, more humanistic, or more ethical. It is being advocated because empirical data show that it is associated with improved physical and mental health outcomes.

We want to make two points about Brody's comments. First, there is an increasing body of research that shows the efficacy of narrative- and relationship-centered care (we shall discuss this work in Chapter 7). Secondly, the phrase "placing the patient's story at the center of the relationship" is used so often today that it is in danger of becoming trite. To honor the patient's story in a meaningful way demands a set of skills that are either lacking, have atrophied, or lie dormant in too many health care professionals. To pay surface attention to the patient's story does nothing to heal the patient or to diminish those barriers which separate patient and physician from an authentic relationship.

Barriers Between Patients and Physicians

Often by the time a person decides to visit a doctor, she has lived with a perceived dysfunction in her "normal" body state. During this period between onset of dis-ease and first contact with a physician, the person's discontinuity with her world begins, as do her physical, cognitive, spiritual, emotional, and financial responses to the separation. There is an attempt to make sense of the illness experience in which the ill person (the narrator) tells or explains to herself (the hearer) what she (the character) is feeling. This *interior narration* is essentially inter-subjective, and hence social. The physician Eric Cassell (86: 33) has conceptualized the multidimensional separation of the person – this interior narration – as "suffering."

> . . . person is not merely mind, merely spiritual, nor subjectively knowable. Person has many facets, and it is ignorance of them that actively contributes to patients' suffering. . . . Suffering occurs when impending destruction of the person is perceived; it continues until the threat of disintegration has passed or until the integrity of the person can be restored . . . suffering can occur in relation to any aspect of the person.

A person carries to the relationship with her physician a state of vulnerability and suffering. In addition, the patient brings meaning to illness events by creating and telling an illness story – a personal narrative that orders and attempts to explain her suffering to herself, to her family, and to her physician.* Kleinman (50: 49) reminds us that the illness story, as with all stories, consists of "plot lines, core metaphors, and rhetorical devices that structure the illness narrative [and] are drawn from cultural and personal models for arranging experiences in meaningful ways and for effectively communicating those meanings." The physician, conditioned by training and routine experiences with disease, suffering, and death, carries to the relationship a different sense of mortality, of explanation, and of the patient's temporality (past, present, and future). Charon (48) has spoken eloquently of these conditions as divides between the sick and the well. Recognizing many conditions that separate physicians and their patients, Charon (48: 22) describes four "urgent" divides:

> *The relation to mortality:* Doctors and patients differ fundamentally in their natural understanding of mortality. Doctors, who know materially about death, accept an actual, present awareness that we are mortal and we will die, while patients, depending on their own personal experiences with illness and death, usually have not developed such concrete realizations. Doctors may look upon death as a technical defeat, whereas patients may see death as both unthinkable and inevitable.
>
> *The contexts of illness:* Doctors tend to consider the events of sickness rather narrowly as biological phenomena requiring medical or behavioral intervention, while patients tend to see illness within the frame and scope of their entire lives.
>
> *Beliefs about disease causality:* Health care professionals and patients can have deeply conflicting ideas about the causes of symptoms and diseases and fundamentally different ways of thinking about those causes. Because beliefs about causality dictate action and ascribe meaning to illness, the treatment, and the ill person, these conflicts can rend care.
>
> *The emotions of shame, blame, and fear:* These emotions, among others, saturate illness and add immeasurably to the suffering it causes. Unless explicitly acknowledged and examined, these emotions and the suffering they cause can irrevocably separate doctor from patient, therefore preventing effective care.

---

* Pellegrino and Thomasma (87) echo these sentiments in their admonition that the vulnerability and dependency of the patient place a special moral obligation on the physician to treat them as a whole person. In the context of a narrative philosophy of medical knowledge, this would translate into there being a special moral obligation to attend to the patient's story of illness and suffering in all of its dimensions, as noted by Cassell.

In the patient story that opens Chapter 1, at least three of these divides influence the relationship between patient and physician and the outcomes of care. First, in terms of *relation to mortality*, the physician sees the treatment he is offering as an alternative to death – as the saving of the patient's life. However, the patient is less conscious of the reality of his own mortality, and is distracted instead by how the treatment has disrupted his present sense of living in the world. Secondly, the *contexts of illness* are quite different between them. For the physician, this patient's kidney disease leads to the need for dialysis, and hence the requirement for the "minor" operation. The context is narrow, being the disease and its treatment. The patient's focus, on the other hand, is directed toward how he will live with the disease of kidney failure, endure the dialysis treatments, and at the same time preserve the continuity of his life story. Finally, this episode demonstrates the pervasiveness of *shame, blame, and fear* in the caregiving enterprise. The patient may be quite ashamed of how his newly dysfunctional hand renders him less a musician, and he fears the loss of productivity and meaning. He likely blames the physician for the disfigurement and functional loss that resulted from his recommendations. The physician may fear being blamed for what he considers to be the "minor" complications that resulted from his well-meaning efforts to prevent major ones.

Interestingly, these same divides serve to separate people from facets of themselves. Each year when I (*JDE*) approach the time for my annual upper endoscopic surveillance for Barrett's esophagus (a precondition of esophageal cancer), I agonize over the possibility of developing cancer and dying from the disease. From the time I call to make the appointment to the day of the procedure (usually a period of a couple of months), I am periodically struck with examining my mortality and the possible disruption of life plans. I believe that, in part, this anxiety is conditioned by the fact that my parents both died from cancer, and one of my closest friends died of esophageal cancer. Having attended his suffering and death, I am aware of the general course of the disease process, and intimately aware of the particulars of my dear friend's suffering over the six-month period from his diagnosis to his death. I find myself attributing various life habits to my diagnosis, temporally linking events to find meaning tinged with cause and blame – too many years filled with spicy foods consumed too hastily while running through 80-hour work weeks. I find during these weeks that I feel more isolated, more distant from friends and loved ones. The disruption and separation are palpable to the closest among them. Ironically, there are also uplifting features. During this period, my meditation practice reminds me of the impermanence of all features of life, and this mindfulness in turn serves to place the material world and personal relationships in order, in a reframed narrative. Just as important, it heightens my awareness that I am in the care of a wise, compassionate and caring healer, one who attends to the connection between my narrative identity and my disease. This mutual honoring and the affiliation that it engenders are what prompt me to travel from Maine to Ohio to be with him and to live in each other's narrative.

Narrative Features of Care and Caring

Charon (48) has postulated five narrative features of clinical practice – temporality, singularity, causality, inter-subjectivity, and ethicality. She argues convincingly and correctly, we believe, that these features help us to better understand the separation of doctors and patients. More importantly, these narrative features provide the agency to decrease the complex distance between patient and physician. As Charon (48: 41) notes, these features align with medical practice.

> A symptom or disease is indeed an event befalling a character, some-times caused by something identifiable, within a specified time and setting that has to be told to another from a particular point of view. However, health care professionals often lack the means to recognize explicitly the temporality within which lives and diseases unfold, to grasp and value the singularity of each person or character, to face both the search for causality and the acknowledgement of underlying contingency in life in general and in disease in particular, and to comprehend the intersubjective and ethical demands of telling one's story and receiving the stories of others.

Temporality

We noted earlier in this chapter the significant role that temporality plays in human experience and action. So, too, it figures prominently in medical practice. "Time", Charon says (48: 44), "is medicine's necessary axis – in diagnosis, prevention, palliation, or cure. Time is, as well, the irreplaceable ingredient in the healing relationship: time to listen, time to recognize, time to care." Health care professionals who practice without this sense of time cause psychological and moral harm to patients. In a qualitative interview study of patient reports regarding preventable problems and harms in primary care (88), for which one of us (*JDE*) was an investigator, 170 discrete harms were reported by patients in their stories of care. An overwhelming 70% of these harms were psychological in character, including anger, frustration, belittlement, and loss of relationship and trust in one's physician. The most common incidents involved breakdowns in the patient–clinician relationship and in access to clinicians. Patients' descriptions of breakdowns in the relationship were dominated by stories of disrespect or insensitivity. Three kinds of problems accounted for over half of the reported breakdowns in access. These were difficulty in contacting the office, delays in obtaining appointments, and excessive office waiting times. Clearly, temporality figures prominently in these perceived harms. Doctors and other health care professionals equipped with a temporal awareness would be sensitive not to commit such patient harms.

Singularity

As we saw in Chapter 1, narrative knowledge focuses on the particulars of person and context. We also saw that, for sociocultural and historical reasons, physicians' sense of the critical importance of singularity to what they do and to the physical and psychological needs of their vulnerable and suffering patients is too often lost. In the study of patient harm discussed above, it is the devaluation of the person's singularity that results in the patients' negative emotions – anger, frustration, and belittlement. Contrary to this situation, when my physician discusses with me (*JDE*) the pathology reports from my endoscopy, he does so not only based on the technical features of the biopsy, but also based on his cognitive and emotional understanding of my uniqueness, my singularity.

Causality

Causation requires a narrative structure in which the presence of a cause is stated and then the effect that it produces is provided. The very notion of plot is based on causation. A plot weaves together a complex set of events to make a coherent story. Plots are a function of the meaning brought to events, and not a function of the events themselves. Plots of illness stories, particularly chronic illness, are dynamic in character. As narrative time moves, the patient and the health care professional engage in a routine characterized by revising interpretations, changing prognoses, judgments, hopes, and therapeutic actions (these complex responsive processes of relating will be discussed in Chapter 3). The resulting story episodes reframe the patient's life in relation to the unknown – the daily, weekly, and monthly surprises. This situation stimulates a cooperative attempt to reframe the narrative plot. This activity – this emplotment – attempts to return coherence to the trajectory of the patient's illness story, and is an effort to continue to find causes and bring order to events. Charon (48: 50) notes:

> Clinical practice is consumed with emplotment. Diagnosis itself is the effort to impose a plot onto seemingly disconnected events or states of affairs. . . . The plot-strong clinician will not stop with the obvious or the evident story line, but will keep looking – generatively, creatively, hopefully in collaboration with the patient – to construct a wide and deep and varied differential diagnosis. This is narrative medicine in practice.

Narrative work is difficult work. Observe how Jack Coulehan works to creatively emplot the care of a "difficult" patient through the use of poetry (89):

The Knitted Glove

You come into my office wearing a blue
knitted glove with a ribbon at the wrist.

You remove the glove slowly, painfully
And dump out the contents, a worthless hand.
What a specimen! It looks much like a regular hand,
warm, pliable, soft. You can move the fingers.

If it's not one thing, it's another.
Last month the fire in your hips had you down,
or up mincing across the room with a cane.
When I ask about the hips today, you pass them off,
so I can't tell if only your pain
or the memory is gone. Your knitted hand
is the long and short of it. Pain doesn't exist
in the past any more than this morning does.

This thing, the name for your solitary days,
for the hips, the hand, for the walk of your eyes
away from mine, this thing is coyote, the trickster.
I want to call, *Come out, you son of a dog!*
and wrestle that thing to the ground for you,
I want to take it by its neck between my hands.
But in this world I don't know how to find
the bastard, so we sit. We talk about the pain.

Jack Coulehan MD

Inter-subjectivity

At its core, the practice of medicine is about an intimate relationship between two individuals. Certainly others are and ought to be involved, but it remains essentially a meeting of two selves. What is the character of this relationship? Carspecken (90: 123), a critical social theorist, in discussing the origin of inter-subjectivity, notes that this idea refers to ". . . prereflective structures that (1) take the existence of other subjects as a given, and (2) constitute experience through the process of position-taking with other subjects . . ." The fundamental importance of inter-subjectivity to life is echoed in another social science tradition, namely symbolic interactionism.* Herbert Blumer (91: 2) summarizes the fundamentals of the tradition in three premises:

> The first premise is that human beings act toward things on the basis
> of the meaning that the things have for them. Such things include
> everything that the human being may note in the world. . . . The
> second premise is that the meaning of such things is derived from,

---

* Inter-subjectivity is echoed in the poem *On Duality* composed by the Buddhist monk Thich Nhat Hahn. This poem can be found at the end of Chapter 1.

or arises out of, the social interaction that one has with one's fellows. The third premise is that these meanings are handled in, and modified through, an interpretive process used by the person in dealing with the things he encounters.

These ideas are important to the understanding of the nature of human relations. Part of our experience of feelings is the understanding that the feeling is not directly available to other subjects, but must be indicated to them through body gestures and words. Thus the inter-subjectivity of objects and feelings is constituted narratively. The implications of the work of social and literary theorists are noted by Charon (48: 53):

> What literary [and social] studies give medicine is the realization that our intimate medical relationships occur in words. Our intimacy with patients is based predominantly on listening to what they tell us, and our trustworthiness toward them is demonstrated in the seriousness and duty with which we listen to what they entrust to us . . . textuality . . . defines the relation. (insertion added)

Trish Greenhalgh describes the phenomenon of inter-subjectivity in medicine when referring to the work of Russian philosopher and linguist Mikhail Bakhtin. According to Greenhalgh (52: 21), ". . . in a Bakhtinian framing of clinical interaction, the role of the clinician is to provide the subjective 'otherness' for an interactional narrative in which the patient will construct, and make sense of, his or her illness narrative."

This position of inter-subjectivity as it is understood by social and literary theorists suggests strongly that physicians need to attend dutifully to the patient's story and to how she tells the story. To do so competently requires a certain set of narrative skills. Narrative skill sets are the subject of Chapter 6.

Ethicality

Taking the idea of inter-subjectivity seriously brings for the physician a moral obligation to honor the patient's story. We have come to understand that there is therapeutic benefit for the patient (and for the practitioner) to be gained from putting into words the meaning of the events that cause disruptions of the body and mind (more will be said about this in Chapters 4, 6, and 7). Because of the patient's vulnerable condition and dependence, the health professional has the responsibility to hear and witness the patient's testimony of suffering and then to act within its context for the benefit of that person (87). Inter-subjectivity is the connection to narrative ethics. Charon summarizes this idea as follows (48: 55):

> Narrative ethics exposes the fundamentally moral undertaking of selecting words to represent what before the words were chosen was

formless and therefore invisible and unhearable. It is the very act of fitting language to thoughts and perceptions and sensations within the teller as to let another "in on it" (that other, the listener . . . now bound intersubjectively . . .) that constitutes the moral act.

Inter-subjectivity connects to virtue ethics as well, as it focuses on the fundamental importance of the practitioner's character. Virtues are taken to be dispositions or acquired qualities that a person habitually brings to her actions in order to achieve some end. In the case of medicine and the patient–physician relationship, that end is the attentive care of a suffering person. Views of narrative ethics implicitly take into account the nature of the moral agent – the clinical practitioner. Health care practitioners, like all human beings, possess a sophisticated reasoning process that is tempered by emotional reactions. These reactions are intimately connected to how we live in the world, and as such they influence our judgments. Virtue ethics recognizes this critical feature of our moral life. Pellegrino and Thomasma (92) have provided a comprehensive treatment of virtue ethics as it connects with the practice of health care. While they argue that there are a number of virtues relevant to the ends of medicine, they offer eight that seem especially relevant – fidelity to trust, compassion, phronesis (practical wisdom), justice, fortitude or courage, temperance, integrity, and self-effacement or altruism. Ethicality then is connected with inter-subjectivity, which in turn is connected with narrative acts committed by people acting in a virtuous manner. Furthermore, the narrative competence of practitioners is facilitated when their actions take place within the context of these virtues.

The nurse and philosopher, Sally Gadow, grounds her work in existential philosophy and brings a dialectic framework to this issue (93–95). Her work resonates with that of Mikhail Bakhtin and Trish Greenhalgh noted earlier. Gadow (93, 95) refers to her approach as *inter-subjective engagement* or *relational narrative* (narrative processes of relating between patient and nurse). She believes that relational narratives are at the core of nursing practice, for they provide a narrative portrait of why nurses practice. Narrative relations between patient and nurse concentrate on the values held, implicitly and explicitly, by the two people. Through a complex process of relating, patient and nurse create a moral narrative that embraces the vulnerability and subjectivity of both as it operates to allow them to live within the context of the present illness moment.

Narrative Competence

There is currently much discussion of narrative competence. We understand competence to be a capacity, an embodied action, sufficient to meet the requirements of the situations in which a person acts (96, 97). We reject the notion that competence is a psychological trait, and rather embrace the position that *what* competence is follows from recognition of *where* it is.* Furthermore, we understand the relationship of skills to competence as one of parts to a whole, where the whole is greater than the sum of its parts. And so while a clinician may have all of the necessary skills for practice, it does not follow that she is competent unless she exercises the wisdom (the virtue of phronesis) to use them (or not) contingent on the requirements of what is best for the care of the patient. Charon (48: vii) reminds us that:

> A medicine practiced with narrative competence will more ably recognize patients and diseases, convey knowledge and regard, join humbly with colleagues, and accompany patients and their families through the ordeals of illness. These capacities will lead to more humane, more ethical, and perhaps more effective care.

What then are the skills that would support narrative competence? In Chapter 6 we discuss and illustrate in detail six skills that are critical to the development and enactment of narrative competence. These are practicing compassionate presence and mindful listening (witnessing and affiliation), exercising moral imagination and expressing clinical empathy, reading and interpreting complex texts (patients), writing reflectively and telling clinical stories (representation), reasoning with stories, and engaging in narrative ethics. As we learn more about narrative practice and its effects, undoubtedly we shall discover additional skills that are important for a wide variety of narrative contexts.

Narrative Contexts

In Chapters 4 and 5, we create a portrait of narrative practice in two types of contexts – contexts of care and contexts of profession and community. The concepts of narrative medicine provide the means to understand the intimate relationship between patient and physician, and to understand the practitioner's self-identity as professional. Here the telling of the patients' stories is a key therapeutic act when attentively witnessed by their physicians. Likewise, when physicians become mindful of their own selves, through reflection and writing, they become aware of how emotional responses to patients affect not only the care of their patients but also their own professional development.

The other type of context we have in mind deals with the stories that health care practitioners tell about their interactions and about what it means to be a health care professional in their time. *Narrative professionalism* is key to understanding where the profession has been, what it is today, and what its possible

---

* Gadow suggests that competence is a function of the professional performance situation when she writes about the nurse–patient relationship as a moral guide to nursing practice. This guide is a relational narrative of the "good" co-constructed by patient and nurse (93, 94). Edwards (98), taking Gadow's idea of relational narrative, argues that this form of narrative leads the nurse to be aware of situations in which to develop a narrative connection with the patient.

futures can be.* Through narrative, the creating and sharing of stories of professional practice, a sense of community happens in a way that can matter to the practice of care and to the development of self. At an even broader level, the collective stories of health care practitioners have been a powerful means of influencing health care policy. Stories at this level present to the public and to policy makers conversations that are important to health policy for local, national, and global communities.

CODA

Throughout this chapter we have been concerned with the turn to narrative as both philosophy and practice that has become central to the intellectual and practical work in a wide variety of professions. In health care, we have argued for the narrative structure of practice within the patient–practitioner relationship. It is now time for us to make explicit the models of relationship that are currently being advocated, and the connection between narrative practice and these models. These become the focus of Chapter 3.

FURTHER ACTIVITIES

1   Readers who are interested in learning more about narrative approaches in health care are encouraged to read the following important works:
   - Brody H. *Stories of Sickness.* 2nd ed. New York: Oxford University Press; 2003.
   - Charon R. *Narrative Medicine: honoring the stories of illness.* New York: Oxford University Press; 2006.
   - Greenhalgh T. *What Seems to be the Trouble? Stories in illness and healthcare.* Oxford: Radcliffe Publishing; 2006.
2   The following websites provide useful information related to narrative medicine:
   - The Centre for Arts and Humanities in Health and Medicine, University of Durham; www.dur.ac.uk/cahhm
   - The Centre for Medical Humanities database, University College London; www.mhrd.ucl.ac.uk
   - The Patient Voices Project; www.patientvoices.org.uk
   - Database of Individual Patient Experience; www.dipex.org.uk
   - Columbia University College of Physicians and Surgeons, program in Narrative Medicine; www.narrativemedicine.org
   - Institute for Medicine in Contemporary Society; www.uhmc.sunysb.edu/prevmed/mns

---

* The concept of *narrative professionalism* was first described by our colleague, Jack Coulehan (99). Jack created this term as a counterforce to the exclusive efforts to conceptualize *professionalism* as a set of quantifiable skills. Narrative professionalism signals the notion that for professionalism to guide behavior, it has to be understood as a meta-narrative, based upon integration of and reflection upon many thousands of stories of the lived experiences of actual health professionals across times and cultures, including direct observations of role-model practitioners.

- Word.doc Narrative Medicine; www.writing.upenn.edu/wh/events/worddoc
- King's College London, Programme in Literature and Medicine; www.kcl.ac.uk/hums/landm
- Centre for Narrative Research; www.uel.ac.uk/cnr/index.htm
- Literature, Arts, and Medicine Database; http://medhum.med.nyu.edu
- The Institute for the Medical Humanities, University of Texas Medical Branch; www.utmb.edu/imh
- Program in Medical Humanities and Health Studies, Indiana University-Purdue University Indianapolis; http://medhumanities.iupui.edu
- Institute for Professionalism Inquiry, Summa Health System; www.summahealth.org (in "Find It" type "Institute for Professionalism Inquiry").

REFERENCES

1 Kreiswirth M. Tell me a story: the narrativist turn in the human sciences. In: Kreiswirth M, Carmichael T, editors. *Constructive Criticism: the human sciences in the age of theory.* Toronto: University of Toronto Press; 1994. pp. 61–87.

2 Ormiston GL, Sassower R. *Narrative Experiments: the discursive authority of science and technology.* Minneapolis, MN: University of Minnesota Press; 1989.

3 Jameson F. *The Political Unconscious: narrative as a socially symbolic act.* Ithaca, NY: Cornell University Press; 1981.

4 MacIntyre A. *After Virtue: a study in moral theory.* Notre Dame, IN: University of Notre Dame Press; 1981.

5 Nussbaum MC. *The Fragility of Goodness: luck and ethics in Greek tragedy and philosophy.* Cambridge, MA: Cambridge University Press; 1987.

6 Ricoeur P. *Time and Narrative. Volume 1.* Chicago, IL: University of Chicago Press; 1984.

7 Ricoeur P. *Time and Narrative. Volume 2.* Chicago, IL: University of Chicago Press; 1985.

8 Ricoeur P. *Time and Narrative. Volume 3.* Chicago, IL: University of Chicago Press; 1988.

9 Rorty R. *Contingency, Irony, and Solidarity.* New York: Cambridge University Press; 1989.

10 Carr D. *Time, Narrative, and History.* Bloomington, IN: Indiana University Press; 1986.

11 Porter DH. *The Emergence of the Past: a theory of historical explanation.* Chicago, IL: University of Chicago Press; 1981.

12 White H. *The Content of the Form: narrative discourse and historical representation.* Baltimore, MD: Johns Hopkins University Press; 1987.

13 Bruner J. *Actual Minds, Possible Worlds.* Cambridge, MA: Harvard University Press; 1986.

14 Bruner J. *Making Stories: law, literature, life.* New York: Farrar, Straus and Giroux; 2002.

15 Crossley ML. *Introducing Narrative Psychology: self, trauma and the construction of meaning.* Philadelphia, PA: Open University Press; 2000.

16 Mishler EG. "Once upon a time . . ." *J Narrative Life History.* 1991; **1**: 101–8.

17 Mishler EG. *Storylines: craft artists' narratives of identity.* Cambridge, MA: Harvard University Press; 1999.

18 Sarbin TR. The narrative as a root metaphor for psychology. In: Sarbin TR, editor. *Narrative Psychology: the storied nature of human conduct*. New York: Praeger; 1986. pp. 3–21.

19 Kreiswirth M. Merely telling stories? Narrative and knowledge in the human sciences. *Poetics Today*. 2000; 21: 293–318.

20 Polkinghorne DE. *Narrative Knowing and the Human Sciences*. Albany, NY: State University of New York Press; 1988.

21 Gee JP. A linguistic approach to narrative. *J Narrative Life History*. 1991; 1: 15–39.

22 Labov W. Speech actions and reactions in personal narrative. In: Tannen D, editor. *Analyzing Discourse: test and talk*. Washington, DC: Georgetown University Press; 1981. pp. 219–47.

23 Linde C. *Life Stories: the creation of coherence*. New York: Oxford University Press; 1993.

24 Ploany L. *Telling the American Story: from the structure of linguistic texts to the grammar of a culture*. Norwood, NJ: Ablex; 1985.

25 Frank AW. *The Wounded Storyteller: body, illness, ethics*. Chicago, IL: University of Chicago Press; 1995.

26 Frank AW. *The Renewal of Generosity: illness, medicine and how to live*. Chicago, IL: University of Chicago Press; 2004.

27 Fox NJ. *Postmodernism, Sociology and Health*. Toronto: University of Toronto Press; 1994.

28 Holstein JA, Gubrium JF. *The Self We Live By: narrative identity in a postmodern world*. New York: Oxford University Press; 2000.

29 Lawrence-Lightfoot S, Davis J. *The Art and Science of Portraiture*. San Francisco, CA: Jossey-Bass Publishers; 1997.

30 Mattingly C, Garro LC. *Narrative and the Cultural Construction of Illness and Healing*. Berkeley, CA: University of California Press; 2000.

31 Felstiner WLF, Abel RL, Sarat A. The emergence and transformation of disputes: naming, blaming, and claiming. *Law Soc Rev*. 1980; 15: 631–54.

32 Symposium on Legal Storytelling. *Michigan Law Rev*. 1989; 87.

33 Cochran L. *Career Counseling: a narrative approach*. Thousand Oaks, CA: Sage; 1997.

34 Csikszentmihalyi M, Beattie O. Life themes: a theoretical and empirical exploration of their origins and effects. *J Hum Psychol*. 1979; 19: 45–63.

35 Savickas M. Career-style assessment and counseling. In: Sweeney T, editor. *Adlerian Counseling: a practical approach for a new decade*. Muncie, IN: Accelerated Development Press; 1989. pp. 329–60.

36 Watkins C, Savickas M. Psychodynamic career counseling. In: Walsh W, Osipow S, editors. *Career Topics: contemporary topics in vocational psychology*. Hillsdale, NJ: Lawrence Erlbaum Associates; 1990. pp. 79–116.

37 Lawrence-Lightfoot S. *The Good High School: portraits of character and culture*. New York: Basic Books; 1983.

38 Noblit GW, Dempsey VO. *The Social Construction of Virtue: the moral life of schools*. Albany, NY: State University of New York Press; 1996.

39 Witherell C, Noddings N. *Stories Lives Tell: narrative and dialogue in education*. New York: Teachers College Press; 1991.

40 Mattingly C. *Healing Dramas and Clinical Plots: the narrative structure of experience*. New York: Cambridge University Press; 1998.

41 Young-Mason J. *Critical Moments: doctor and nurse narratives and reflections.* Bloomington, IN: First Books; 2003.

42 Darbyshire P. Understanding caring through arts and humanities: a medical/ nursing humanities approach to promoting alternative experiences of thinking and learning. *J Adv Nurs.* 1994; **19:** 856–63.

43 Darbyshire P. Lessons from literature: caring, interpretation, and dialogue. *J Nurs Educ.* 1995; **34:** 211–16.

44 Younger JB. Literary works as a mode of knowing. *Image J Nurs Sch.* 1990; **22:** 39–43.

45 Sakalys JA. Restoring the patient's voice: the therapeutics of illness narratives. *J Holist Nurs.* 2003; **21:** 228–41.

46 Mullan F, Ficklin E, Rubin K. *Narrative Matters: the power of the personal essay in health policy.* Baltimore, MD: Johns Hopkins University Press; 2006.

47 Brody H. *Stories of Sickness.* 2nd ed. New York: Oxford University Press; 2003.

48 Charon R. *Narrative Medicine: honoring the stories of illness.* New York: Oxford University Press; 2006.

49 Greenhalgh T, Hurwitz B. *Narrative-Based Medicine: dialogue and discourse in clinical practice.* London: BMJ Books; 1998.

50 Kleinman A. *The Illness Narratives: suffering, healing, and the human condition.* New York: Basic Books; 1988.

51 Launer J. *Narrative-Based Primary Care.* Oxford: Radcliffe Medical Press; 2002.

52 Greenhalgh T. *What Seems to be the Trouble? Stories in Illness and Healthcare.* Oxford: Radcliffe Publishing; 2006.

53 Iser W. *The Act of Reading: a theory of aesthetic response.* Baltimore, MD: Johns Hopkins University Press; 1978.

54 Dosse F. *Empire of Meaning: the humanization of the social sciences.* Minneapolis, MN: University of Minnesota Press; 1999.

55 Hiley DR, Bohman J, Shusterman R. *The Interpretive Turn: philosophy, science, culture.* Ithaca, NY: Cornell University Press; 1991.

56 Rorty R. *The Linguistic Turn: recent essays in philosophical method.* Chicago, IL: University of Chicago Press; 1967.

57 Simons HW. *The Rhetorical Turn: invention and persuasion in the conduct of inquiry.* Chicago, IL: University of Chicago Press; 1990.

58 Turner M. *The Literary Mind.* New York: Oxford University Press; 1996.

59 Foss L. *The End of Modern Medicine: biomedical science under a microscope.* Albany, NY: State University of New York Press; 2002.

60 Rossi EL. *The Psychobiology of Mind–Body Healing.* New York: Norton; 1986.

61 Maturana H, Varela FS. *The Tree of Knowledge: the biological roots of human understanding.* Boston, MA: Shambala; 1992.

62 Damasio A. *The Feeling of What Happens: body and emotion in the making of consciousness.* London: Heinemann; 1999.

63 Golden L, Hardison OB, translators. *Aristotle's Poetics: a translation and commentary for students of literature.* Tallahassee, FL: Florida State University Press; 1990.

64 Kearney R. *On Stories: thinking in action.* New York: Routledge; 2002.

65 Ricoeur P. Life in quest of narrative. In: Wood D, editor. *On Paul Ricoeur: narrative and interpretation.* London: Routledge; 1991. pp. 20–33.

66 Taylor C. *Sources of the Self: the making of modern identity.* Cambridge, MA: Harvard University Press; 1989.

67 Waitzkin H. *The Politics of Medical Encounters: how patients and doctors deal with social problems*. New Haven, CT: Yale University Press; 1991.

68 Rosenwald GC, Ochberg RL, editors. *Storied Lives: the cultural politics of self-understanding*. New Haven, CT: Yale University Press; 1992.

69 Skultans V. Narratives of the body and history: illness in judgment on the Soviet past. *Sociol Health Illn*. 1999; **21**: 310–28.

70 Rimmon-Kenan S. The story of 'I': illness and narrative identity. *Narrative*. 2002; **10**: 9–27.

71 Brockmeier J, Carbaugh D, editors. *Narrative and Identity: studies in autobiography, self and culture*. Philadelphia, PA: John Benjamins Publishing Company; 2001.

72 Ricoeur P. *Oneself as Another*. Chicago, IL: University of Chicago Press; 1992.

73 Frank AW. The rhetoric of self-change: illness experience as narrative. *Sociol Q*. 1993; **34**: 39–52.

74 Eakin P. *How Our Lives Become Stories: making selves*. Ithaca, NY: Cornell University Press; 1999.

75 Holstein J, Gubrium J. *The Self We Live By: narrative identity in a postmodern world*. New York: Oxford University Press; 1999.

76 Carib I. Narratives as bad faith. In: Andrews M, Day Sclater S, Squire C, Treacher A, editors. *Lines of Narrative: psychosocial perspectives*. London: Routledge; 2000. pp. 64–74.

77 Sacks O. *The Man Who Mistook His Wife for a Hat and Other Clinical Tales*. New York: Summit Books; 1985.

78 Brody H. *Stories of Sickness*. New Haven, CT: Yale University Press; 1987.

79 Hunter KM. *Doctor Stories: the narrative structure of medical knowledge*. Princeton, NJ: Princeton University Press; 1991.

80 Nelson HL, editor. *Stories and Their Limits: narrative approaches to bioethics*. New York: Routledge; 1997.

81 Mattingly C. *Healing Dramas and Clinical Plots: the narrative structure of experience*. Cambridge: Cambridge University Press; 1998

82 Charon R. The ethicality of narrative medicine. In: Hurwitz B, Greenhalgh T, Skultans V, editors. *Narrative Research in Health and Illness*. London: BMJ Books; 2004. pp. 23–36.

83 Bury M. Illness narratives: fact or fiction? *Sociol Health Illn*. 2001; **23**: 263–85.

84 Leopold N, Cooper J, Clancy C. Sustained partnerships in primary care. *J Fam Pract*. 1996; **42**: 129–37.

85 Roter DL, Hall JA, Kern DE *et al*. Improving physicians' interviewing skills and reducing patients' emotional distress: a randomized clinical trial. *Arch Intern Med*. 1995; **155**: 1877–84.

86 Cassell EL. *The Nature of Suffering and the Goals of Medicine*. New York: Oxford University Press; 1991.

87 Pellegrino ED, Thomasma DC. *A Philosophical Basis of Medical Practice: toward a philosophy and ethic of the healing professions*. New York: Oxford University Press; 1981.

88 Kuzel AJ, Woolfe, SH, Gilchrist V *et al*. Patient reports of preventable problems and harms in primary care. *Ann Fam Med*. 2004; **2**: 333–40.

89 Coulehan J. *The Knitted Glove*. Troy, ME: Nightshade Press; 1991.

90 Carspecken PF. *Four Scenes for Posing the Question of Meaning and Other Essays in Critical Philosophy and Critical Methodology*. New York: Lang; 1999.

91 Blumer H. *Symbolic Interactionism.* Englewood-Cliffs, NJ: Prentice-Hall; 1969.

92 Pellegrino ED, Thomasma DC. *The Virtues in Medical Practice.* New York: Oxford University Press; 1993.

93 Gadow S. Relational narrative: the postmodern turn in nursing ethics. *Sch Inq Nurs Pract.* 1999; **13:** 57–70.

94 Gadow S. Ethical narratives in practice. *Nurs Sci Q.* 1996; **9:** 8–9.

95 Romyn DM. The relational narrative: implications for nurse practice and education. *Nurs Philos.* 2003; **4:** 149–54.

96 LaDuca A. The structure of competence in health professions. *Eval Health Prof.* 1980; **3:** 253–88.

97 Engel JD, Sayers S, LaDuca A *et al. Competence in Clinical Dietetics.* Chicago, IL: Center for Educational Development, University of Illinois Medical Center; 1980.

98 Edwards SD. *Philosophy of Nursing: an introduction.* New York: Palgrave; 2001.

99 Coulehan J. I witness, I serve: medicine as community. In: *Proceedings of the Fourth Humanism and the Healing Arts Conference. Institute for Professionalism Inquiry.* Akron, OH: Summa Health System; 2006.

CHAPTER 3

The Patient–Practitioner Relationship

Practically every development in medicine in the post World War II period distanced the physician and the hospital from the patient and community, disrupting personal connections and severing bonds of trust. . . . By the 1960s the two had moved so far apart that one could have asked a lay audience about the last time they spoke to a physician and had their clothes on, and they would have been unable to remember an occasion.

David J Rothman (1: 127)

The recent growth in patient-centered care is a response to the narrowness of medicine's contextualization. Patient-centered care is a conceptual and clinical movement, arising both in the United States and the UK, that emphasizes the patient's perspectives and desires throughout all aspects of health care.

Rita Charon (2: 27)

- INTRODUCTION
- FACTORS THAT SEPARATE PATIENTS AND PRACTITIONERS
- PATIENT-CENTERED AND RELATIONSHIP-CENTERED CARE
- COMPLEX RESPONSIVE PROCESSES OF RELATING

KEY IDEAS

- There are both structural (practice location, specialization, and pace of work) and non-structural (psychological and intellectual) elements of the health care system that divide patients and practitioners.
- In part, these divides are the legacy of biomedical models of care.
- Alternative models of the patient–practitioner relationship have been advocated as a means of alleviating these divides and providing more humane and effective health care.
- These alternative models – biopsychosocial, patient-centered, and relationship-centered – all place the patient's illness story at the center of a caring relationship. Some models, such as relationship-centered care, also value the contextual uniqueness of both patient and physician.
- At a practical level, the theory of complex responsive processes of relating provides a social psychological explanation for the unique connections between relationship-centered care and narrative health care.

INTRODUCTION

In Chapter 1 we discussed how the theory and practice of modern medicine is a reflection of a struggle for cultural authority and upward social mobility. Remember that from the late 1700s until the early 1900s the relationships among medical education of that period, the dramatic influence of Scottish, English, French, and German medical practice and science, and the reform of the university system in the USA all became important contextual factors in framing the modern biomedical model. While critically successful in improving some aspects of health, the biomedical model came under increasing criticism as an all-encompassing model for health care delivery and research.* Although these critiques have been rich in proposing a variety of alternatives, they are in agreement that the model of biomedicine essentially separates mind and body so that the patient becomes objectified and has no self that is centrally important to the clinical encounter. We have seen that the general thrust of these critiques is to reconnect mind and body and to return the patient as a reflective and reflexive self to the center stage of clinical care. Central to movement of the patient to center stage is the place of the patient's story or narrative.

Subsequently, in Chapter 2, we examined the narrative turn in several disciplines and professions. Along with that turn, we saw the critical importance of narrative identity to patients' selfhood and the character of suffering as represented in illness stories. Throughout Chapter 2 we showed how narrative

---

* Current representations of the biomedical model in the form of practice informed by evidenced-based medicine (EBM) certainly provide a necessary, although not sufficient, element of quality health care. EBM as progeny of the biomedical model suffers all of the limitations, all of the philosophical and practical flaws of the parent [see Henry SG, Zaner RM, Dittus RS. Moving beyond evidenced-based medicine. *Acad Med.* 2007; **82:** 292–7.]. The current challenge for health care is to create a community that values narrative truth and integrates narrative practice with appropriate versions of EBM.

structures are an inherent part of clinical practice and are a window on the patient–practitioner relationship.

Here in Chapter 3 we more fully examine the nature of the relationship between patient and practitioner. We discuss how alternative models of the relationship seek to restore the central place of narrative in the transactions between practitioners and their patients. Following this, we explore recent interdisciplinary work that provides a theoretical and practice foundation for models of relationship-centered care. Finally, we explore how narrative medicine and the practitioner's narrative competence connect with and constitute the character of this relationship.

FACTORS THAT SEPARATE PATIENTS AND PRACTITIONERS

Historians of modern medicine such as Rothman (1) and Shorter (3), who study the various types of relationships between patients and their practitioners in different time periods, have noted a variety of structural and non-structural elements that serve to divide practitioners from their patients. Charon (2) highlighted four different kinds of divides – relation to mortality, contexts of illness, beliefs about disease causality, and emotions of shame, blame, and fear. The non-structural separations that Charon addresses are essentially psychosocial and intellectual in character. We shall now examine the structural elements that serve to separate practitioners from their patients.

Focusing on structural changes in US health care following World War Two, Rothman (1) notes that the most significant change for the relationship between patient and physician was the demise of the routine house call. This move made the lives of physicians more efficient, and provided greater income. By bringing patients to the office or hospital, practitioners could examine more patients in far less time. This change removed the patient from a familiar environment and deprived the physician of a more intimate and nuanced knowledge of the whole patient and her environment. Both symbolically and literally, patients and physicians were distanced.

The increased specialization and sub-specialization following the war years served to train physicians in particular organs and organ systems. The more they narrowed their study, the easier it was to lose sight of the patient as a whole person. Speaking about this period, Shorter (3: 194) notes that "In a major postmodern development, the style of medicine as a whole has become the style of one of its specialty branches: the specialty of *internal medicine*, which is everything from the neck to the navel." Internists, in the beginning, were consultants and would see other physicians' patients who had grave clinical problems. However, as Shorter (3) argues, the internist's role widened extensively due to the drug revolution in the 1950s, and internists found themselves acting as personal physicians. To this expanded role, the internist brought a style that valued the intense pursuit of diagnosis and the treatment of biophysical disease with drugs or surgery. For many internists this tended to result in a devaluation of the person's illness story. It was not a serendipitous event that the practice of medical interviewing by internists moved from the taking of conversational medical histories to the use of structured "yes–no" questions related to specific regions of the body. This development was reinforced with the move to efficiency noted above. The subsequent depersonalization of clinical care, due to these structural changes, dramatically decreased both the patient's opportunity for storytelling and expressions of suffering, and the practitioner's reflective understanding of her patient and herself in relation to her patient's life.

Another significant structural change is the increased pace and almost frenetic rhythm of contemporary practice. Time is functional for so many important matters in health care, and yet the time for practitioners to exercise narrative skills such as compassionately attending to their patients and mindfully reflecting on their practices has diminished severely. The narrative structure of this dimension both for the individual practitioner and for medicine as a community is the subject of Chapters 4, 5, and 6. For now, suffice it to say that time restrictions, while real, might be re-storied (re-emploted) so that they could bring clinicians and patients closer to one another, rather than separating them.

The resulting loss of focus on the patient as person has caused many observers within and outside medicine to develop and advocate a different model of patient–practitioner relationship – one that is patient- or relationship-centered and fundamentally based on narrative competence and practice.

PATIENT-CENTERED AND RELATIONSHIP-CENTERED CARE

The nature of the patient–physician relationship has been described from antiquity to modern and postmodern times (3–8). One thing that is clear in the descriptions of medical practice over time is that there has been a decline in the centrality of narrative to the health care encounter (5, 6). As psychological and structural divides have become more pronounced, there has been a concomitant loss in the appreciation of narrative practice. The various postmodern critiques of the nature of the patient–physician relationship may be seen as attempts to philosophically and practically reframe the clinical encounter as the core relationship between two people, one of whom seeks attentive compassionate care from the other.

Engel's (9) advocacy for a biopsychosocial model and Balint's (10) creation of the idea of "patient-centered medicine" were early attempts to describe the belief that each person has to be understood and treated as a unique human being. This idea was further developed by Stewart and Brown and their colleagues (11, 12) along the lines of a patient-centered clinical method that embraced six separate but related components:

1 pursuing the illness as well as the disease experience
2 being sensitive to the whole person
3 cooperatively deciding treatment and management

4 discussing disease prevention and health promotion
5 exploring common ground
6 recognizing structural constraints in the clinical setting, such as time and available resources.

Advocacy for this reframed model of the patient–practitioner relationship tacitly criticized and thus called into sharp relief the characteristics of existing models.

Roter and Hall's (6) work on types of patient–practitioner relationships provides a clear analysis of key variables framing the relational context. They base their conceptualization on the expression of power and dynamics of negotiation between patient and practitioner.* This analysis is reproduced in Table 3.1.

Table 3.1 Types of Doctor–Patient Relationship (6: 26)

Patient Control	Physician Control	
	Low	High
Low	Default	Paternalism
High	Consumerism	Mutuality

As noted by Roter and Hall (6), *default* occurs when the patient's and physician's expectations of the relationship are in conflict. When this conflict cannot be negotiated, one or both people decide to leave the relationship. Communication failures result in dysfunctional and failed relationships that represent frustration and emotional turmoil for both participants. This circumstance often sets the stage for anger and malpractice (16).

Paternalistic forms of patient–practitioner relationships are those in which the physician dominates the encounter in all respects, and devalues the patient's illness perspective. This structural arrangement allows for the smooth functioning of what are thought to be relationships typical of the modern period (6, 17). This type of relationship was the cornerstone of Parsons' structural-functionalism theory of the patient–physician relationship (14). In this model, the patient must seek help and comply with the treatment regimen. The doctor's role is to exercise complete authority in an autonomous society, and provides the patient with nurturing and support from the physician (6).

Medical consumerism in the USA represents relationships in which patients set the agenda and goals of the encounter. This form of relationship has been stimulated by a move from curative to preventive health care, as well as a related and broader social movement that shifts the role of person from patient to

---

* Roter and Hall recognize that these ideal models are based on theoretical work by Talcott Parsons (13, 14) in the 1950s, and contrasting work by Elliot Freidson (15) in the 1970s. At the core of these bodies of work is the idea of conflict between patient and physician, and between professional authority and patient autonomy. It is beyond the scope of our work to detail this historical and philosophical debate. Interested readers are referred to the work of Parsons and Freidson listed in the References section at the end of this chapter.

consumer (18). Such a relationship changes the roles of patient and physician by shifting their relative power status, decreasing physician authority and increasing patient autonomy. Care is centered on the preferences and values of the patient. Extreme forms of this type of relationship can be misunderstood and misinterpreted as honoring patient-centeredness on the part of some clinicians. In this "patient-centric" model, the physician functions as a technical advisor, thus limiting the positive health effects of her clinical authority as well as her expression of affect and emotion (6).

Roter and Hall (6: 27) suggest that encounters characterized by *mutuality* change the social relationship between patient and practitioner:

> In this model, each participant brings strengths and resources to the relationship on a relatively even footing. Inasmuch as power in the relationship is balanced, the goals, agenda, and decisions related to the visit are the result of negotiation between partners; both the patient and the physician become part of a joint venture. Medical dialogue is the vehicle through which the patient's values are explicitly articulated and explored.

More importantly, the mutuality model reframes the construct of *relationship* and places it at center stage. The construct of mutual relationship signals both specific tasks and values for patient and practitioner – a search for mutual personhood. Here relationship is framed by a complex process of respectful listening and responding to each other's values, vulnerabilities, strengths, and expertise.

Given these models of patient–physician relationship, an interesting question concerns the place of patients' illness narratives within them. The work of British sociologist Mike Bury suggests some interesting connections. Bury (19) notes that, historically, in Britain in the seventeenth and eighteenth centuries an aristocratic physician was expected to pay close attention to the patient's illness story, develop an intimate relationship with the patient, and suggest treatment through procedures that restored the body's equilibrium. With the ascent of biomedicine, hospitals, and laboratory procedures, the importance of the patient's story diminished and, in Roter and Hall's terms, the patient lost control, and the physician gaining higher control adopted (with the tacit consent of the patient) a paternalistic role in the relationship. However, a variety of social and political forces operating through time have reopened space for the centrality of the patient's story. Bury (19) attributes the renewed attention to patients' stories to several factors. First, there has been a relative decline in infectious diseases, which were a primary context and foundation for the biomedical model, and a dramatic increase in chronic and degenerative diseases. Secondly, with increased costs of hospital care, there has been a renewed emphasis on primary care as a way of controlling health costs. Associated with primary care is sensitivity to the patient's illness story. Thirdly, there has been an increased

move toward democratic ideals and open society (supported by rapid information exchange) in late modern cultures, sensitizing both physicians and patients
to relationships of mutuality in Roter and Hall's terms.

The work of Roter and Hall, along with that of Bury, foreshadowed the next
development in ways of constructing the moral relationship between patient and
physician. It was a careful examination of the philosophy and practice of patient-
centered care that led the Pew-Fetzer Task Force on Advancing Psychosocial
Health Education in 1992 to suggest the next iteration toward a philosophy of
medical care (20). The group developed an explicitly values-based foundation
for the work of health care practitioners, known as *relationship-centered care (RCC)*.
This model of care is predicated upon four related principles:

1 health care relationships ought to include characteristics of personhood as
  well as roles
2 health care relationships must recognize the important and central place
  of affect and emotion
3 mutuality is a hallmark of all health care relationships
4 there is a moral foundation to RCC.[*]

In reframing patient-centered care as RCC, Beach and colleagues (22)
broaden the idea of relationship to include relationships between clinician and
colleagues, clinician and community, and clinician and self. Before moving on
to explore each of the principles mentioned above, we should note that this
broad notion of *relationship* is similar to that postulated in 2001 by Charon (23)
in her discussion of the four central narrative situations of concern to narrative
medicine, which we shall examine in Chapters 4 and 5. Thus we find essentially
the same proposal for an extended notion of relationship coming from two
different but related movements – narrative medicine and relationship-centered
care. Now let us turn to an examination of each of the four principles of RCC.

Relationship and Personhood

RCC explicitly values the contextual uniqueness of both patient and practitioner.
Unlike other models, the practitioner in RCC is conceptualized as one who
remains aware of her emotional reactions to patients, and monitors her
behavior, given this awareness. Beach and colleagues (22) point out that the
idea of practitioner-as-person has been underdeveloped in typical accounts of
patient-centered care. They write (22: S4):

> In addition to the explicit recognition that clinicians bring their
> personhood into the encounter, RCC emphasizes the importance of

---

[*] The Institute of Medicine's report (21: 49) cites as one of the aims for improving the US health care
system a patient-centered approach to care. The report lists six dimensions of care: ". . . (1) respect
for patients' values, preferences, and expressed needs; (2) coordination and integration of care; (3)
information, communication, and education; (4) physical comfort; (5) emotional support – relieving
fear and anxiety; and (6) involvement of family and friends."

authenticity, in the sense that clinicians should not, for example, simply act as if they have respect for someone; they must also aim actually to have (internally) the respect that they display (externally).

Affect and Emotion

In RCC, it is the emotional presence of the clinician that provides support to the patient. RCC rejects the idea of detached concern prevalent in biomedical models of relationship and clinical training (24). Developing and expressing clinical empathy is a critical component of RCC. Communication of emotions by the practitioner in the relationship with a patient demonstrates caring and often influences healing. In addition, it gives permission to the patient to express her emotions to the practitioner.

Mutuality

In RCC, unlike previous models of relationship, both patient and practitioner are encouraged to exchange and create stories together. Each gets to know the other, and in doing so each influences the character of the other. This mutuality increases the likelihood of positive outcomes for the patient and a growth in virtuous behavior for the practitioner.

RCC as Moral Concept

Duggan and colleagues have examined the question of whether there is a moral imperative to follow a patient-centered care model (25). Their analysis applies equally well to relationship-centered care. In a close examination of three prominent ethical traditions – consequentialist, deontological, and virtues-based – they conclude (25: 274):

> Using consequentialist reasoning, patient-centered care is morally required, on account of the empirical evidence that it leads to improved outcomes for patients. Using deontological reasoning, patient-centeredness may be justified because many of the features of patient-centered care align with important ethical norms and principles, for example, respect for persons, shared decision-making, and the responsibility to care for particularly vulnerable patients. Finally, patient-centeredness also encompasses an element of virtues-based ethics in its insistence that physicians possess a moral capacity for self-reflection and a desire to better understand and adopt those attitudes and dispositions that positively influence their own behaviors.

These three widely held ethics positions all arrive at a similar viewpoint – that relationship-centered care has a moral foundation.

In summary, RCC represents the latest development in a series of moves to turn the patient–practitioner relationship from its potentially dehumanizing form within the biomedical model to a form that is sensitive to the subjectivity of both patient and practitioner. This was the purpose of RCC's predecessors – patient-centered care and biopsychosocial medicine. Although RCC offers a philosophy and an approach to care, it has not specified the nature of relationships and how they work.

Recently, Anthony Suchman, an internist who trained under George Engel, has creatively outlined a theoretical underpinning for RCC based on work in *complex responsive processes of relating* (26).

COMPLEX RESPONSIVE PROCESSES OF RELATING

Ralph Stacey, psychoanalyst and complexity theorist, has integrated the work of sociologist Norbert Elias on social processes, the theory of symbolic interactionism of George Herbert Mead, and a particular strand of complexity theory from the natural sciences to explain how patterns of relating and associated meaning-making are continuously created as individuals interact (27, 28).* Because Stacey integrates three complex idea systems, complex responsive processes of relating (CRPR) is a very rich and multifaceted theory, full explication of which is beyond our present purposes. The interested reader is directed to the collective works of Stacey and his colleagues listed in the Further Activities section at the end of this chapter.† We do, however, want to focus on one aspect of CRPR that is particularly relevant to relationship-centered care and narrative health care, namely self-organizing patterns of meaning and relating.

Relying on Shotter's work (30) concerned with the realities of conversations, Stacey notes (27: 130):

> The central proposal is that human interaction is essentially a process in which people account to each other, negotiate with each other, in a collaborative process in order to "go on" together. . . . Coherence and order are reproduced and potentially transformed in a self-organizing process that is the meshing together of individual actions. This is an approach that does not distinguish between the level of the individual and the level of the social, but sees them as different aspects of the same phenomenal level. . . . There is no split between theory and practice either, because the theory, or explanation of action, is precisely what is being negotiated in that action.

---

* We raise two observations here. First, much of Stacey's work relies upon a dynamic approach to understanding stories in context, and this position is reminiscent of earlier work of Elliot Mishler. Secondly, there are two strands of complexity theory. One is based on a Kantian view that causality in nature unfolds an existing ontology. This is known as *formative teleology*. The other strand of complexity theory, the one that Stacey follows, is based on the work of Hegel and interpreted by George Herbert Mead. It assumes that the future or reality is under continuous construction. It is neither fixed nor permanent. This is referred to as *transformative teleology*.

† We would also note that Shapiro (29) in 1993 wrote about a similar idea within the practice of family medicine, namely that narrative is a reciprocal relational experience.

Stacey (27) points out that this approach to human communicative interaction has been informed by extensive work conducted in multiple disciplines, namely ethnomethodology (31, 32), conversational analysis (33, 34), and social constructionism (29, 35). Based on this body of work, Stacey (27: 130) notes that the common features of patterned human communicative interaction are ". . . mutual expectations of associative response; turn-taking sequences; sequencing, segmenting and categorizing actions; rhetorical devices." Witness these dynamic features in the following conversation between a physician and his patient.*

Dr Gardner: You said you had headaches. Are they in the same place as before?

Mrs Flowers: Yes, same place, same feeling, only more often. Does that matter?

Dr Gardner: I'm not sure yet. Have you had any difficulty with your vision?

Mrs Flowers: No.

Dr Gardner: Any nausea?

Mrs Flowers: No. Well, when I drank the pickle juice there was some.

Dr Gardner: Pickle juice? Now that has a lot of salt in it and it's not good for your hypertension. Why did you do that?

Mrs Flowers: My mother told me that I need it because I have high blood and that is why I have headaches and pressure.

Dr Gardner: And just what does the pickle juice do?

Mrs Flowers: Well, it thins the blood and reduces the pressure and the aches in my head.

Dr Gardner: After all these years I've known you, I didn't know about that remedy. Well, we'll need to talk more about this and I think we should have your mother come by when we do. Would that be possible and would it help?

Mrs Flowers: I thought you might say something like that. She should hear what you have to say about her remedy that she got from her mother. I can just hear her now.

Dr Gardner: OK. In the meantime the salt isn't good for your hypertension. It will make it worse, and that is likely to give you more headaches. So please don't drink any more pickle juice.

In this interaction, we can hear the associative responses offered by the physician and the patient as they take turns allowing the other to complete the sequences

---

* This conversation between Dr Gardner and Mrs Flowers is a modification of a longer exchange originally recorded in Arthur Kleinman's book, *The Illness Narratives: suffering, healing and the human condition* (New York: Basic Books; 1988. p. 133).

of their thoughts, while at times using instructive and directive forms of talk (rhetorical devices). The very features of this interaction facilitate coherence and pattern in people's ongoing communicative actions. However, as noted by Stacey (27), while the patterning produces coherence and stability, it also allows for change to be initiated. The potential for new understandings resides in those moments that strike people. Dr Gardner is struck by the folk remedy of pickle juice, and this variation in what he knows interrupts the ongoing flow and spontaneous exchange of the encounter. This conscious interruption encourages him to begin to explore this unique variation and, in so doing, potentiates changes in him and Mrs Flowers, and thus changes in his relationship with Mrs Flowers.

Stacey (28: 75) argues that as people act communicatively with each other, each simultaneously acts communicatively with herself:

> These silent private conversations . . . have exactly the same features as public vocal conversations . . . minds are associative, with one thought or voice silently triggering another thought or voice. . . . The same sequencing of turn taking is evident as first one aspect of oneself and then another takes turns, makes turns, to participate in role plays . . . some thoughts have a voice and others are denied or repressed . . . the same kinds of rhetorical devices are in evidence in one's silent conversation . . . striking moments call forth responses from oneself.

In Chapter 2, we spoke of this phenomenon as *interior narration*, and it is represented in the conversation between Mrs Flowers and Dr Gardner.

> Dr Gardner: After all these years I've known you, I didn't know about that remedy. Well, we'll need to talk more about this and I think we should have your mother come by when we do. Would that be possible and would it help?

> Mrs Flowers: I thought you might say something like that. She should hear what you have to say about her remedy that she got from her mother. I can just hear her now.

Both seem to be having a silent conversation with themselves that in a meaningful way is interacting with their public conversation and creating the pattern of that interaction.

Stacey goes on to draw an analogy between the patterning effect of communicative interaction and narrative. In this regard, there is striking synergy between his ideas and those of the phenomenologist Carr, described in the previous chapter. Here we see the multiple theoretical viewpoints converging to explain the same phenomenon. Stacey (28: 76) writes:

> . . . those collective and individual histories reproduced in the living present of communicative action are extending those histories into

the future. This points to the narrative-like structuring of human experience. It is not simply that people are telling each other stories or that narrative is simply an alternative type of knowledge. The turn-taking, responsive relating of people may be thought of as forming narrative at the same time as that narrative patterns moral responsibility and turn taking. In other words, the experience of the living present, like the past, is structured in narrative-like ways. It is in the micro interaction of their turn-taking conversations that people are perpetually constructing the narrative pattern of the living present and thus the future.

Here a word needs to be said about the phrase "narrative-like." Stacey (28: 76) clarifies this:

> This kind of "narrative told" must be distinguished from the narrative-like processes that are narrative-in-its-making. Interaction . . . evolves as narrative-like themes that normally have no single narrator's perspective. Beginnings and endings are rather arbitrary, and there are many plots emerging simultaneously. The narrative told is retrospective, while the narrative-in-its-making is currently emerging in the living present. The former is inevitably linear while the latter is intrinsically nonlinear.

Stacey's point about nonlinearity is based on the contention that self-organizing patterns of communicative action occur in the course of iterative reciprocal interactions. Suchman states (26: S41–2):

> Iterative reciprocal interactions are the hallmark of nonlinear dynamics (complexity) in which there is no equilibrium state and patterns can shift unpredictably. . . . Another important property of nonlinear interactions is known as the amplification of small differences. In the course of an iterative reciprocal interaction, a slight difference – say a new phrase or slightly different behavior – may elicit a new response that carries the difference further and itself elicits a response that elaborates the difference further still. In just a few cycles of interaction, the small difference can be amplified into a new, transformative pattern. . . . One final implication of nonlinear dynamics is that the emergence of novel patterns of meaning or relating requires both diversity and responsiveness in the interaction. When little diversity is exhibited (perhaps because participants do not believe it is welcomed), there are fewer serendipitous differences to spark cascades of change.

In the encounter between Mrs Flowers and Dr Gardner we see an illustration of just such a slight difference iteratively generating a new relational pattern.

Dr Gardner: Any nausea?

Mrs Flowers: No. Well, when I drank the pickle juice there was some.

Dr Gardner: Pickle juice? Now that has a lot of salt in it and it's not good for your hypertension. Why did you do that?

Mrs Flowers: My mother told me that I need it because I have high blood and that is why I have headaches and pressure.

Dr Gardner: And just what does the pickle juice do?

Mrs Flowers: Well, it thins the blood and reduces the pressure and the aches in my head.

Dr Gardner: After all these years I've known you, I didn't know about that remedy. Well, we'll need to talk more about this and I think we should have your mother come by when we do. Would that be possible and would it help?

Mrs Flowers: I thought you might say something like that. She should hear what you have to say about her remedy that she got from her mother. I can just hear her now.

Interestingly, in Stacey's theorizing, we see an argument from the perspective of CRPR that is completely consistent and sympathetic with the arguments in Chapter 2 (particularly those of Carr) regarding narrative identity.

To recapitulate, Stacey's theory of complex responsive processes of relating provides a theoretical underpinning for relationship-centered care. CRPR highlights the micro dynamics of human communicative actions and constructs these actions as a relational process driven by self-organizing patterns of meaning. It centrally locates and values attentive responsiveness and diversity as critical to moral relationships. Communicative action constructs both individual minds and social realities. Stacey (28: 78) summarizes his position eloquently:

> In communicative interaction, people actively respond to each other, and in so doing their experiences are patterned in narrative-like forms. Human experience is story-like. In their relational communication people are constructing intricate narratives and abstract–systematic frameworks. When they reflect on what they have been doing, on what they are doing and on what they hope to do, they select aspects of these dense narratives . . . to tell stories . . . in order to account for what they are doing and make sense of their worlds. In the process their very identities, individually and collectively, emerge.
>
> My proposition, then, is that all human relationships, including the communicative action of a body with itself, that is mind, and the communicative actions between bodies, that is social, are story lines and propositions constructed by those relationships at the same time

those story lines and propositions construct the relationships. They are all complex responsive processes of relating that can be thought of as themes and variations that recursively form themselves in bodily interaction.

CRPR is a way of making sense of what the term *relationship* means in the phrase *relationship*-centered care. And since the meaning of relationship is narrative in nature, the theory and practice of narrative medicine connects intimately with the theory and practice of relationship-centered care. At a theoretical level these two concepts complement one another, and narrative medicine at the level of narrative competence provides the practical means for enacting relationship-centered care. It is narrative medicine as it is represented in the narrative relationships of patient and practitioner, practitioner and self, practitioner and colleagues, and practitioner and community that we explore in Part 2. Following this, we move on to the critical issue of what constitutes narrative skills, and how they can be developed in the service of informed and nuanced versions of relationship-centered care.

FURTHER ACTIVITIES
Readers who are interested in learning more about the history of patient–physician relationships and complex responsive processes of relating are encouraged to read the following texts:

- Shorter E. *Doctors and Their Patients: a social history.* New Brunswick, NJ: Transaction Publishers; 1991.
- Lain Entralgo P. *Doctor and Patient.* New York: McGraw Hill; 1969.
- Stacey RD. *Complex Responsive Processes in Organizations: learning and knowledge creation.* New York: Routledge; 2001.
- Stacey RD. *Complexity and Group Processes: a radically social understanding of individuals.* New York: Brunner-Routledge; 2003.
- Beach MC, Inui T, for the Relationship-Centered Care Research Network. Relationship-centered care: a constructive reframing. *J Gen Intern Med.* 2006; **21:** S3–8.
- Stewart M, Brown JB, Weston WW *et al. Patient-Centered Medicine: transforming the clinical method.* 2nd ed. Oxford: Radcliffe Medical Press; 2003.

REFERENCES
1 Rothman DJ. *Strangers at the Bedside: a history of how law and bioethics transformed medical decision making.* New York: Basic Books; 1991.
2 Charon R. *Narrative Medicine: honoring the stories of illness.* New York: Oxford; 2006.
3 Shorter E. *Doctors and Their Patients: a social history.* Piscataway, NJ: Transaction Publishers; 1991.
4 Lain Entralgo P. *Doctor and Patient.* New York: McGraw Hill; 1969.

5 Roter DL. The enduring and evolving nature of the patient–physician relationship. *Patient Educ Couns.* 2000; **39:** 5–15.

6 Roter DL, Hall JA. *Doctors Talking with Patients/Patients Talking with Doctors: improving communication in medical visits.* 2nd ed. Westport, CT: Praeger; 2006.

7 Szasz TS, Hollender MH. A contribution to the philosophy of medicine: the basic model of the doctor–patient relationship. *Arch Intern Med.* 1956; **97:** 585–92.

8 Szasz TS, Knoff WF, Hollender MH. The doctor–patient relationship and its historical context. *Am J Psychiatry.* 1958; **115:** 522–7.

9 Engel G. The need for a new medical model: a challenge for biomedicine. *Science.* 1977; **196:** 129–36.

10 Balint E. The possibilities of patient-centered medicine. *J R Coll Gen Pract.* 1969; **17:** 269–76.

11 Stewart M, Brown JB, Weston WW *et al. Patient-Centered Medicine: transforming the clinical method.* 2nd ed. Oxford: Radcliffe Medical Press; 2003.

12 Brown JB, Stewart M, Weston WW, editors. *Challenges and Solutions in Patient-Centered Care: a case book.* Oxford: Radcliffe Medical Press; 2002.

13 Parsons T. *The Social System.* Glencoe, IL: The Free Press; 1951.

14 Parsons T. The sick role and the role of the physician reconsidered. *Millbank Q.* 1975; **53:** 257–78.

15 Friedson E. *Professional Dominance.* Chicago, IL: Aldine Press; 1970.

16 Levinson W, Roter DL, Mullooly J *et al.* Doctor–patient communication: a critical link to malpractice in surgeons and primary care physicians. *JAMA.* 1997; **277:** 553–9.

17 Emanuel EJ, Emanuel LL. Four models of physician–patient relationship. *JAMA.* 1992; **267:** 2221–6.

18 Reeder LG. The patient-client as a consumer: some observations on the changing professional–client relationship. *J Health Soc Behav.* 1972; **13:** 406–12.

19 Bury M. Illness narratives: fact or fiction. *Soc Health Illn.* 2001; **23:** 263–85.

20 Pew-Fetzer Task Force on Advancing Psychological Health Education. *Health Professions Education and Relationship-Centered Care.* San Francisco, CA: Pew Health Professions Commission; 1994.

21 Committee on Quality of Health Care in America, Institute of Medicine. *Crossing the Quality Chasm: a new health system for the 21st century.* Washington, DC: National Academy Press; 2001.

22 Beach MC, Inui T, for the Relationship-Centered Care Research Network. Relationship-centered care: a constructive reframing. *J Gen Intern Med.* 2006; **21:** S3–8.

23 Charon R. Narrative medicine: a model for empathy, reflection, profession and trust. *JAMA.* 2001; **286:** 1897–902.

24 Halpern J. *From Detached Concern to Empathy: humanizing medical practice.* New York: Oxford University Press; 2001.

25 Duggan PS, Geller G, Cooper LA *et al.* The moral nature of patient-centeredness: is it "just the right thing to do"? *Patient Educ Couns.* 2006; **62:** 271–6.

26 Suchman AL. A new theoretical foundation for relationship-centered care: complex responsive processes of relating. *J Gen Intern Med.* 2006; **21:** S40–44.

27 Stacey RD. *Complex Responsive Processes in Organizations: learning and knowledge creation.* New York: Routledge; 2001.

28 Stacey RD. *Complexity and Group Processes: a radically social understanding of individuals.* New York: Brunner-Routledge; 2003.

29 Shapiro J. The use of narrative in the doctor–patient encounter. *Fam Syst Med.* 1993; **11:** 47–53.

30 Shotter J. *Conversational Realities: constructing life through language.* Thousand Oaks, CA: Sage Publications; 1993.

31 Garfinkel H. *Studies in Ethnomethodology.* Englewood Cliffs, NJ: Prentice-Hall; 1967.

32 Goffman E. *Forms of Talk.* Philadelphia, PA: University of Pennsylvania Press; 1981.

33 Sacks H. *Lectures on Conversations.* Oxford: Blackwell; 1992.

34 Boden D. *The Business of Talk: organizations in action.* Cambridge: Polity Press; 1994.

35 Shotter J, Katz AM. Hearing the patient's 'voice': toward a social poetics in diagnostic interviews. *Soc Sci Med.* 1996; **46:** 919–31.

PART 2

Professional Performance Situations and Narrative Importance

Part 2 carefully examines the place of narrative in four situations originally identified in the work of Rita Charon – patient and practitioner, practitioner and self, practitioner and colleagues, and practitioner and community. In each situation the power and utility of story to better understand who one is and what is transacted in complex encounters are examined and illustrated. In Chapter 4, two of these situations are framed within the core notion of caring for patients and for oneself. Chapter 5 examines the two more macro situations and frames them within the broader social organization of colleagues and communities.

CHAPTER 4

Narrative Contexts of Care

Telling stories is as basic to human beings as eating. More so, in fact, for while food makes us live, stories are what make our lives worth living. They are what make our condition human.

Richard Kearney (1: 3)

Researchers may be uneasy addressing this "soft" subject, but it is critical to the viability of any health system, whatever its shape or character, and central to public trust and confidence. It represents the heart of what patients want from health care – enhancement of their sense of well-being, relief from their suffering.

Lennart Fredriksson and Katie Eriksson (2: 3)

KEY IDEAS

- Illness disrupts a person's life narrative, making that person vulnerable. Such an ill person seeks, through a relationship with a caregiver, to reconstruct the life narrative in ways that offer healing.
- Many models exist to describe the special features of the patient–caregiver relationship. A narrative approach to that relationship enables the fully competent caregiver to provide care within all such models, balancing logico-scientific with narrative competence.
- Narrative medical practice serves many functions, including transformation of caregivers to broader ways of seeing and caring, better self-understanding for patients, and greater potential for healing.
- Illness stories construct two landscapes – the landscape of action and the consciousness landscape. Narrative medical practice requires that caregivers become competent to provide care informed in both landscapes.
- In narrative medical work, moral imagination involves the ability to understand one's own values and biases as a caregiver, openness to the particularity of the patient's experience, an attempt to fully understand the lived experience from the patient's perspective, and co-construction by caregiver and patient of a new narrative of healing.
- Placing the patient's needs ahead of one's own – the obligation of altruism – is a central ingredient of narrative competence.
- Narrative competence requires that caregivers fully develop their skills in self-awareness, reflective learning, and practice. Educators are obligated to ensure that there is sufficient time and space for such development in all areas of health professions education.

INTRODUCTION

The opening chapter of *Stories Matter*, edited by Rita Charon and Martha Montello, presents a conversation with Jerome Bruner in which he comments on medicine's *coming around* to the importance of narrative. He observes that being rational initiates the dehumanizing process (3). Bruner's observation about rationality calls to mind a highly anthologized poem by Wallace Stevens (4: 73), entitled "Six Significant Landscapes", the sixth stanza of which is quoted below:

> Rationalists wearing square hats,
> Think, in square rooms,
> Looking at the floor,
> Looking at the ceiling.
> They confine themselves
> To right-angled triangles.
> If they tried rhomboids,

> Cones, waving lines, ellipses –
> As, for example, the ellipse of the half-moon –
> Rationalists would wear sombreros.

Clearly Stevens is neither condemning the rational, nor suggesting the abandonment of rational thinking. He is simply offering, through the use of the metaphor of the half-moon, a new way of looking at the world – a broader imagining. If, as Bruner suggests, rationality can be seen in medical work as a manifestation of dehumanization, then a narrative turn in that work just might offer a way to provide the broader way of seeing that Stevens implies.

Bruner (3: 8) adds emphasis to this point, stating:

> The fact of the matter is that if you look at how people actually live their lives, they do a lot of things to prevent their seeing the narrative structures that characterize their lives. Mostly, they don't look, don't pause to look. Not even when they are doctors and are supposed to be concerned with the life-and-death stories of their patients.

This *not looking* can be a powerful force in separating us from *other*. Yet we find meaning in connection and in narratives that connect us. Rainer Maria Rilke (5: 98) exposes the fallacy of attempting to separate ourselves from others in the following poem.

Love Song

How can I keep my soul in me, so that
it doesn't touch your soul? How can I raise
it high enough, past you, to other things?
I would like to shelter it, among remote
lost objects, in some dark and silent place
that doesn't resonate when your depths resound.
Yet everything that touches us, me and you,
takes us together like a violin's bow,
which draws one voice out of two separate strings.
Upon what instrument are we two spanned?
And what musician holds us in his hand?
Oh sweetest song.

Rainer Maria Rilke

In the previous chapter we highlighted some of the forces which have served to distance people seeking care from the professionals who provide it. We mentioned the structural changes in the nature of medical practice that have exacerbated this distancing, including increased specialization and subspecialization, and an emphasis on clinical productivity that reduces available time spent in the clinical encounter. In this chapter and the next one, echoing the description by Rita Charon (6) of the four complex *narrative situations*, we shall examine the place of narrative in four domains – patient and practitioner, practitioner and self, practitioner and colleagues/profession, and practitioner and community.* In each situation the power and utility of story to better understand who we are and what is transacted in complex encounters will be examined. The first two dimensions will be discussed in Chapter 4, and the latter two in Chapter 5.

We begin this chapter with descriptions of the narrative features of the patient and of the caregiver, and their relationship. We then discuss the functions of narrative in caregiving relationships, and the landscapes within these illness narratives. The importance of caregiver competence in these landscapes is elaborated. We conclude the discussion on the patient–caregiver domain by defining moral imagination in narrative medical practice, and finally by discussing the challenge of altruism in that work. We conclude Chapter 4, moving to the practitioner–self domain, by discussing the caregiver self as an important tool in narrative work, and how that caregiver self is influenced by the educational process. Finally, we discuss the critical importance of self-awareness and reflective practice in narrative medicine.

NARRATIVE IN THE PATIENT–PRACTITIONER DIMENSION
The Patient

The person seeking care from the health care practitioner often approaches this relationship with some degree of brokenness or vulnerability, and in search of healing. Characteristically, such an individual has experienced disruption of what Bruner (7) describes as the *canonical* baseline state of affairs in her life, typically as a result of illness or injury. The narrative of this person's life takes a sudden turn and she finds herself in uncharted territory, in a new lifeworld. She approaches the caregiver with hope for redress in order that the state of affairs in her life might be restored, and that the plot of her life story might be reconstituted. And while the healing sought would most ideally include her whole person (body, mind, and spirit), the training of health professionals focuses on cure (biological restoration of homeostasis).

Healing in its broadest sense has been described as the *ends of medicine* by Pellegrino and Thomasma (8: 52–3). They suggest that:

> . . . the ends of medicine are ultimately the restoration or improvement
> of health and, more proximately, to heal, that is, to cure illness and

---

* In the same year that Charon published her work, Greenhalgh published a piece in which she spoke of four important situations for narrative in medicine, namely stories for exploring "otherness", stories for promoting the imagination, stories for critical reflection on professional practice, and stories as a research tool. There is resonance between the ideas of Charon and Greenhalgh (see Greenhalgh T. Storytelling should be targeted where it is known to have greatest added value. *Med Educ.* 2001; **35**: 818–19.)

disease, or, when this is not possible, to care for and help the patient to live with residual pain, discomfort, or disability.

They further elaborate that patients and physicians, acting together as *moral agents*, are motivated to assure that these ends for a particular patient are *right and good*, not just technically, but from a moral perspective as well. In the search for healing, the patient seeks to return to wholeness and a normal life so far as that is possible (8). Such a definition of healing derives from the root of the word relating to a concept of wholeness, and, as Donovan (9:16) notes, ". . . involves restoring function, maintaining function, or at the very least, regaining the sense of balance and the integration of meaning and living." The disintegrating force of crisis or illness in one's life must be addressed in ways that restore the integrity of one's living, as well as its meaning.

The disruption of one's life course that leads one to seek health care can lead to suffering, an experience characterized by Cassell (10: 33) as occurring ". . . when an impending destruction of the person is perceived; it continues until the threat of disintegration has passed or until the integrity of the person can be restored in some other manner." This conception of integrity of the person lies at the center of the illness narrative, and all efforts to heal must be at some level focused on its preservation or restoration. In order for the illness narrative to be understood in ways that might facilitate healing, and in order that the suffering might best be addressed, the person must be understood. And while cautioning that a person cannot best be understood by a reductionistic approach – that is, by reducing such a person to individual components or parts – Cassell (10) presents a *simple topology of person* that is useful in reminding us of the complexity of such understanding. He points out that every person has:

- personality or character
- a past
- a family
- a cultural background
- roles
- relationships with others
- relationship with self
- a political nature
- things one does
- a degree of unawareness
- regularity of behaviors
- a body
- secret dimensions
- a perceived or imagined future
- transcendency or spirituality.

The complexity of personhood depicted in Cassell's topology serves as a poignant reminder that the healer who seeks to restore the integrity of personhood for the sufferer must somehow come to appreciate the potential for suffering and disruption to impact on any of the numerous dimensions that comprise the whole person. Likewise, breaches in any, and often many, of these dimensions may need to be addressed to truly achieve the ends of medicine. Consciousness of the damaged personhood of the sufferer may be the healer's most important tool for, as Cassell (10: 44) eloquently points out, "The human body may not have the capacity to grow another part when one is lost, but the person has."

One additional characteristic of the patient that is worthy of mention is the *de facto* vulnerability which every ill person experiences. This vulnerability stems from what Davis (11: 29), citing previous work by Pellegrino, describes as ". . . the 'existential inequality' of the patient–physician relationship born of the ineradicable 'fact of illness.'" This fundamental characteristic of the ill self arises from a number of forces. First, there is *disorder*. It arises as illness or injury disrupts the understood course of the person's well life. This disorder may evolve into chaos for a time as the person grapples with the experience of illness. In many instances the patient is able to manage some degree of control over this disorder, but in certain instances the illness experience may deteriorate into what Arthur Frank (12) describes as a *chaos narrative*, whose plot is characterized by a lack of control and the absence of hope for improvement.

Illness also creates *fear*, as the patient experiences a sense of unknowing, particularly with regard to both the meaning of one's life and one's future. Illness, as the nursing scholar Jurate Sakalys (13: 229) has described, becomes:

> . . . an ontological assault, acting through a nexus of disruptive events: human power to act is compromised, the body becomes foreign and is medicalized, productive functioning is lost, and relationships and expectations for the future change.

The ill person has difficulty imagining what may come next.

A third force leading to vulnerability is the *isolation* that illness creates. By virtue of what is *wrong* with them, patients become separated from their usual environments of home, relationships, and work. An example can be seen in an exercise we assign to our third-year medical students which asks them to write imaginatively in the voice of one of their patients. One student described an aging physician struggling with falls and dementia who, from his hospital bed, sees the residents and students in the hallway making rounds and asks, "Am I still part of that team?" She represented his disconnectedness, by virtue of his illness, not only from the medical team that symbolized his former work, but also from the human team as well.

Fourthly, the ill person experiences a *loss of privacy*, as illness prompts the need for exposure and analysis that often uncover body parts, as well as, in fact, life parts, that were previously held as private and one's own. The person's body and story are transformed into *specimen* and *case* and placed on display, to be understood generally, documented, and classified, rather than respected and protected.

Finally, there is *depersonalization*. The erosion of personal identity is a well-known consequence of illness as caregivers attempt to generalize a particular person's illness experience into broad taxonomies of disease. Medical work is aimed at classifying and theorizing in ways that mean the particular becomes generalizable, so that a diagnosis can be made, and a treatment plan concocted. What results is a shift of attention from what the patient experiences to what the caregiver interprets of such experiences, so that a *theory* of that patient's illness can be devised. Robert Coles (14: 21) laments the risks of such an approach, warning that ". . . in our self-consciousness as . . . theorists we lose sight of human particularity." The patient becomes the disease, is often referred to by bed number or diagnosis rather than by name, and thus, as Sakalys (13: 228) points out, ". . . patienthood is experienced as a disintegration of self, as an interruption of one's biography, and as a silencing of one's voice." As we discussed in Chapter 1, the risk involved in mistaking our abstractions or generalizations of a particular patient's illness is what Whitehead (15) referred to as the *fallacy of misplaced concreteness*.

The Practitioner

Hope abounds that people who choose to work as health care professionals are motivated by a fundamental concern for and desire to help others. Once they have been trained and credentialed, caregivers bring great power to their relationships with patients. More than one dictionary includes *magical powers* as one definition of medicine, underscoring the scope of the power to heal. By virtue of becoming members of a profession, caregivers possess highly specialized knowledge and training that they are expected to apply in service to others, namely the sick. Just as a patient's vulnerability creates inequality in the patient–caregiver relationship, so does this *power* of the caregiver.

Pellegrino and Thomasma describe *temperance* as a critically important virtue used by clinicians to counterbalance the forces of medical power. They stress that physicians are obligated to carefully weigh the appropriateness of offering, for example, available scientific and technologic treatment options in a particular patient's care by tempering their appetites for such treatments in ways that assure that decisions are made purely for the patient's *good* (8). Such a virtuous approach, in their view (8: 120), resists ". . . the temptation to 'play God'", a temptation which may lead to ". . . inappropriate judgments about either the patient's values or the patient's quality of life . . ." being made.

Howard Brody (16) has described the physician's power as having three components:

- *Aesculapian power*, deriving from the specialized training in the profession of medicine
- *charismatic power*, arising from the physician's own personal attributes and interpersonal abilities

- *social power*, resulting from the status of the physician granted by a society in return for upholding medicine's contract with that society.

These elements of a physician's power, which may apply similarly in nursing and other caregiving professions, grant a degree of authority* and autonomy in medical work. Such power elicits trust on the patient's part that the caregiver will use these powers in service to the patient. With such power comes the professional's responsibility to honor and maintain that trust.

Armed with these professional powers, caregivers can be described as bringing certain tendencies to the caregiving relationship. As mentioned previously, one of these should be genuine concern for the welfare of others. Friedson (18) distinguishes the *clinical mind* from that of the scientist by virtue of five specific attributes:

1 a tendency toward *action*, where doing something, even with little hope of a successful outcome, is valued above doing nothing
2 *belief in the work* as something which is good and worthwhile
3 *pragmatism*, favoring results over theory
4 *trust in personal experience*, giving power to the clinician's instincts and subjectivity as shaped by experience
5 an ability to deal with *uncertainty*, allowing for a broader range of possibilities than pure science might offer.

Friedson (18: 170) states further:

> In assuming responsibility for the practical action he takes, the practitioner also assumes a degree of vulnerability, for while he may gain the gratitude due the miracle worker, he may also gain the reproach due the man who fails to work miracles. In assuming responsibility for virtually any concrete and practical action, one also assumes a risk and thus is always vulnerable to reproach, legal and otherwise. It seems appropriate that the clinician should feel a certain righteousness and pride in being willing to assume responsibility, and a certain defensiveness and paranoia about the risk of reproach.

These tendencies on the part of the clinician predict, Friedson argues, a certain individualism, or an affinity for the particular rather than the universal. "Thus", he claims (18: 170–1), ". . . a rather thoroughgoing particularism, a kind of ontological and epistemological individualism is characteristic of the clinician." Given the clinician's interest in action and practical results, as well as subjectivity based upon his own experiences, Friedson (18:170–71) states that he may come to:

---

* The concept of cultural authority in medicine as described by Paul Starr (17) is discussed in Chapter 1.

. . . rely on the authority of his own senses, independently of the general authority of tradition or sciences. . . . In part because he is so absorbed in and isolated by his own work, he is likely to see and evaluate the world more in terms of his own experience than in terms of what authorities tell him.

This affinity for the particular in relation to a drive toward generalized knowledge is further characterized by Kathryn Montgomery (19: 46–7), who writes that, for clinicians, "The interpretive reasoning required to understand signs and symptoms and to reach a diagnosis is represented in all its situated and circumstantial uncertainty in narrative." She argues that the clinical judgment so critical to the physician's competence goes beyond the reasoning of scientists, and functions as what she describes as *narrative rationality*. Physicians manage a database of scientific knowledge and are required to interpret those data in the context of a particular patient's experience. As Montgomery (19: 47) posits, physicians ". . . must negotiate the fit between the organizing principles of their professional worldview and specific problematic situations. . . . Narrative, thus, is essential to thinking and knowing in clinical medicine."

Friedson's original descriptions of the *clinical mind* were written just under 40 years ago, and it is worth considering whether anything has changed since then. First, it can be argued that while science and technology have advanced dramatically, the fundamental characteristics of the clinical caregiver may have evolved very little. The affinity for action may in fact be stronger as more and more *things to do* have become available to caregivers. Secondly, the extent to which caregivers believe in and value the work that they do as good and worthwhile is likely multiplied by the ever improving outcomes of clinical work. Thirdly, pragmatism continues to reign in modern medicine, and the modern-day push toward evidence-based medicine signals even greater emphasis on empirical results rather than plausible theories. Fourthly, while caution is clearly taught regarding subjectivity in clinical practice, traditional clinical education continues to be taught, both in medicine and in nursing, in ways that value the wisdom and first-hand experience of senior clinicians balanced with the *evidence* published in texts and current literature. Finally, it seems clear that despite continued advances in scientific knowledge, the potential for uncertainty persists. Paradoxically, as we have become better at predicting and measuring outcomes, the unpredictable in medicine has become more pronounced.

The assertion that the clinical mind is one possessed of an *ontological and epistemological individualism* makes the implications for the clinician's work in the patient–caregiver relationship significant (18). We would suggest that the movement toward narrative practice, in which a caregiver comes to understand, interpret, and operate in the lived experience of another, may not be particularly natural. Designing educational modalities aimed at allowing learners to nurture and develop their empathic skills beyond their own individual perspectives becomes obvious. These educational approaches are the subject of Chapter 6.

The Patient–Practitioner Relationship

In this section we want to extend as well as reinforce the ideas discussed in Chapter 3, because they are at the core of all health care encounters. We begin by returning to the thoughts of Jerome Bruner. Narrative, as described by Bruner (7: 16), ". . . deals with the vicissitudes of human intentions." Such *vicissitudes* – defined as dramatic shifts in circumstances or fortunes – are at the heart of the patient–caregiver encounter, since patient and caregiver so often meet at a crisis point in the patient's story. Bruner (7) describes stories, or *lifelike narratives,* as beginning with a *canonical or legitimate steady state* which is disrupted, creating crisis. The state of crisis then requires some form of redress, allowing either for a return to the original steady state or for the development of some new or modified steady state. In medicine, illness and/or injury are just such disruptions, and patients meet caregivers while in need of redress. These disruptions in steady state, in Bruner's formulation, are not dissimilar to what we described in Chapter 2 in the work of Rimmon-Kenan (20), who describes illness as a disruption to the coherence of one's life narrative or sense of self, or to Arthur Frank's (12) description of *narrative wreckage.* Frank identifies storytelling, the essence of narrative work, as a *way out* of the wreckage.

The patient–caregiver relationship is often born out of this sort of critical turn in the unfolding of a person's life, which by necessity creates a relationship that is characteristically asymmetric and complex. What is transacted in that relationship is the very essence of medicine, as Cassell (10: 69) states:

> Through the relationship it is possible, given the awareness of the necessity, the acceptance of the moral responsibility, the understanding of the problem and the mastery of the skills, to heal the sick; to make whole the cured, to bring the chronically ill back within its fold, to relieve suffering, and to lift the burdens of illness.

Much has been written about this special relationship, and its history and evolution over time have been widely studied. Clearly it is not a relationship among equals – there is inequality of knowledge, power, and obligation. Yet each participant needs the other. Each has a purpose in the relationship, each has needs to be met, and each has ways of being in the relationship which will influence the outcomes of what gets transacted within it.

Pellegrino and Thomasma (8) outline five features of the patient–physician relationship which, taken together, construct the moral landscape of medical work. The first, which we have already described, is that of *inequality,* where the patient is vulnerable and the caregiver possesses special powers. This inequality places particular obligation on the caregiver to act in the best interests of the patient. The second feature is the *fiduciary nature* of the relationship and the trust that patients place in the competence and motivations of the caregiver. The third feature is the special nature of medical decisions having both *technical* and *moral* dimensions. Decisions must be technically and morally sound – correct for the patient's particular malady, and at the same time *for the patient's good.* The fourth feature is medical *knowledge,* and how it grants the caregiver a special invitation into the life of the patient, and how it must be used exclusively in service to the suffering. Finally, the *moral complicity* of physicians is in serving patients as the ultimate guardians of their well-being.

In Chapter 3 we discussed the work of Roter and Hall (21) in characterizing patient–physician relationships along a continuum of patient and physician control. A number of other models of the patient–caregiver relationship have been proposed in an attempt to further characterize the roles of each participant, and the manner in which they work together. Psychiatrists Thomas Szasz and Marc Hollender (22: 586–7) described three basic models as follows:

- Activity–Passivity: The patient remains passive and the caregiver *does* something to the patient.
- Guidance–Cooperation: The sick person seeks help, and the caregiver guides the patient to action; the patient cooperates with the recommendation for care.
- Mutual Participation: The patient and caregiver participate together to satisfy each other's needs.

This concept of mutual participation, as with Roter and Hall's (21) *mutuality,* places the relationship at the very center of medical work. Interestingly, at the time when their work was published in the mid-1950s, Szasz and Hollender (22) described the mutual participation model as essentially non-applicable in medicine. Its allusions to a partnership model of care seemed out of place in an era of medical paternalism and a balance of relational power that was shifted heavily in favor of the physician. More recently, the physician scholars Ezekiel and Linda Emanuel (23) have described four models of the patient–physician relationship:

- Paternalistic Model: The physician determines what is best for the patient, and the patient is expected to accept this determination.
- Informative Model: The physician informs the patient of options, the patient chooses, and the physician carries out the patient's choice.
- Interpretive Model: The physician attempts to understand the patient's values, and then works with the patient to make choices in line with these values.
- Deliberative Model: The physician educates the patient about health-related values, and the patient and physician then work together to develop a plan of action which best reflects those values.

Yet another perspective on theoretical models for the patient–caregiver relationship is that of Michael Yedidia (24), a researcher at the Rutgers Center for State Health Policy. Yedidia characterizes the relationship in three broad categories that are consistent with those discussed in Chapter 3. The first category includes *functionalist* models in which the caregiver, by virtue of her training and expertise, knows what is best for the patient, is trusted by virtue of that expertise, and for whom emotional involvement is seen as a potentially negative force upon objective, expert decision making. Next are *patient-centered* models, which emphasize the continued importance of caregiver expertise, but direct that expertise at the needs of the patient so that patient autonomy becomes central to how care is provided and how decisions are made. Here again, emotionality plays no role, and the patient–caregiver connection is grounded in what the patient wants in the light of the caregiver's expert advice. Finally, there are *relationship-centered* models, in which each participant comes as an *authentic self*, and a relationship is developed through shared understanding. In this construct, caregivers and patients come as individual *persons* rather than in particular *roles*, and the mutual purpose that connects them becomes a force for healing. Here, emotions are described as essential to healing and *authenticity*. The genuine interaction of individuals is seen as central to the goals of the work transacted within the relationship.

In all of these models, the obligations of the participants, their autonomy, and their roles vary considerably. Each model has value in certain circumstances, and each has potential benefits as well as the risk of harm. The way in which these models and their relative application in medicine have evolved reflects a movement from what Brody (16) describes as the *old ethics*, where doctors decide what is good for the patient, to the *new ethics*, steeped in patient autonomy and at the other end of the spectrum from paternalism.

The shift toward placing relationship at the center of what transpires between patient and caregiver underscores the value of narrative as a framework for understanding. It also addresses contemporary criticisms of medicine as depersonalized and non-humanistic, and shifts from what McArthur and Moore (25) characterize as a *commercial culture* of service provision to a more *professional culture*, fundamentally motivated to serve the sufferer above all else. The increasing interest in narrative is reflected in a burgeoning literature. A growing number of scholars, educators, and clinicians appear to be developing into what Rita Charon describes as a *federation* of like-minded individuals committed to narrative competence as essential to clinical competence.* Health professions education must attend to its relevance and value in contemporary health care.

It is important to recognize that for all of these depictions of the patient–caregiver relationship (those by Roter and Hall, Szasz and Hollender, Emmanuel and Emmanuel, Yedidia, Beach and colleagues, and others not described here), the constructs are theoretical. In reality, caregiving relationships are often transacted in ways that cut across the categories or distinctions outlined within such constructs. In any given circumstance, features of one model may be preferred over those of another, or a patient may be best served through

---

* Personal communication, May 2007. Charon's comments are presented in greater detail in Chapter 8.

approaches that intersect more than one model. For example, an unconscious trauma patient is completely reliant upon the autonomous and expertise-driven decisions and actions of the caregiver, so even paternalistic care has a place in medicine. In chronic illness, or in palliative care as observed by Yedidia (24), the relationship moves to a place of greater importance, and its participants are more likely to rely upon how they come to relate to one another, how they feel in relating, and how they bring their authentic selves to the enterprise.

Proposing a narrative model for the caregiving relationship, then, is fraught with the same theoretical and practical limitations and serves to demonstrate how a models-based understanding is best described as overlapping rather than distinctive patterns. Nonetheless, it is worth comparing narrative medicine with other models. To consider a narrative model for the patient–caregiver relationship, it is important to build upon the theoretical work described in Chapters 2 and 3 (especially our discussion of complex responsive processes of relating) in order to understand what narrative is, to explore its fundamental characteristics, to assess its value, and to know how it can or should be applied in medical work.

Brody (26: 13) writes that "Suffering is produced and alleviated by the meaning that one attaches to one's experiences. The primary human mechanism for attaching meaning to particular experiences is to tell stories about them." The patient, then, arrives at the patient–caregiver relationship in search of meaning through the construction of stories. The caregiver is invited to hear these stories in a generous way, and to work with the teller to co-construct new stories. The subsequent work of the relationship is transacted in those stories and their continued telling and re-telling, all aimed at the *ends of medicine* – to provide healing. Nursing scholars Lennart Fredriksson and Katie Eriksson (2: 4) write that ". . . suffering is understood, ontologically, as a drama with three acts: confirmation of suffering, being in suffering, and becoming in suffering." If agreement could be reached that these are indeed the three acts, then a narrative model for the caregiving relationship would require that the caregiver be capable of serving the sufferer in ways which confirm the suffering, bear witness to it in a sharing way, and then assist in an ongoing narrative construction which leads to a new reality of meaning and restoration of self for the sufferer.

In her book *What Seems to be the Trouble?*, Trisha Greenhalgh (27) discusses differing viewpoints from the academic literature on just what narrative is. She cites the *referential perspective*, in which narrative is simply a person's storytelling – a telling of what happened. Also mentioned is the *transformative perspective*, a storytelling aimed at *changing* what happened – as, for example, in the formation or reframing of the storyteller's identity. Finally, she describes the *performative perspective*, where the storytelling is the action in itself. Narrative in medicine, we would argue, presents the value of all three of these approaches at various times and in varied proportions.

Greenhalgh (27) further states that narratives possess defining characteristics which include *chronology, characters, context, emplotment,* and *trouble.* The events within a story are played out over a time course, involve multiple individuals in addition to a protagonist, are situated in a culture or environment particular to the central character, unfold in patterns and turns which give the story meaning, and perhaps most importantly, center on some crisis (as in Bruner's construct) or so-called Aristotelian *peripeteia* – defined as a breach in the expected course of events – which triggers the story's unfolding. Charon (28: 114–26) describes a similar set of ". . . five aspects of the narrative text – frame, form, time, plot, and desire", each of which can enrich a reader's experience within a particular narrative. As is demonstrated in the opening story in Chapter 1, caregivers in a narrative model of the patient–caregiver relationship will be most effective if they are capable of understanding their patients' narratives with some appreciation of how each of these characteristics gives shape to their patients' lived experiences of illness. This point will be discussed in greater detail in Chapters 6 and 7.

An understanding of the various models for the caregiving relationship is instructive. Understanding how these relationships lead to healing, or fail to do so, has implications for the education of caregivers, and for their ongoing development and sustenance. More importantly, however, it should be stated that the fully competent caregiver must be able to provide care within all of these theoretical frameworks, and must be sensitive to the situational appropriateness of any given framework for a particular patient. Thus, if caregiver education emphasizes logico-scientific preparation and competence without such emphasis on narrative work, caregivers may be left short-handed, with patients in search of better healers.

Narrative Matters

Physiologist and neuroscientist Felice Aull (29) discusses how Charon's model of narrative medicine fits with other meta-narratives of science and medicine, and in so doing adds to our exposition of why narrative is important in caring for others. Aull acknowledges that a narrative approach gives recognition and meaning to the *emotional and existential status* of ill people. She describes the value of caregivers coming to know, through narrative practice, who and how they are and what they bring as a result to the work of caring for sufferers. Finally, she (29: 290) cites the importance of outing the ". . . contingent and constructed nature of medical knowledge" in the context of broadening caregivers' understanding of the uncertainties of medicine. This argument offers hope, she continues, that such understanding will result in greater realism on the part of caregivers about what really can or should be done for a particular patient with a particular lived experience of illness. These arguments support the *broader knowing* that results from imagining the completeness of Stevens' half-moon mentioned earlier in this chapter. They also speak to the importance of a *shared knowing* that results from the mutual participation of patient and caregiver in the patient's illness narrative.

Narratives have many components, as we reviewed earlier, and they also serve many functions. Richard Kearney (1: 128–56), drawing upon the writings of Aristotle, has elaborated upon the *enduring functions of storytelling*, including *plot (mythos)*, *re-creation (mimesis)*, *release (catharsis)*, *wisdom (phronesis)*, and *ethics (ethos)*. Although all of these functions arise from illness narratives, we believe that some are particularly relevant to the power of narrative medicine. Mimesis has been discussed earlier in Chapter 2, so we begin here with the concept of catharsis.

Kearney's (1: 137) description of *catharsis* as ". . . the idea that stories 'alter' us by transporting us to other times and places where we can experience things *otherwise*" highlights the transformative power of operating in our patients' illness narratives. In experiences with particular patients' narratives, a caregiver can learn to provide better care and become a better care provider. And as caregivers *experience things otherwise*, they are afforded the opportunity ". . . to be sufficiently *involved* in the action to feel that it matters." Just as such involvement in a work of fiction evokes empathy for its characters, the connections that occur between caregiver and patient in the patient's illness narrative strengthen caregiver empathy.

Kearny describes *phronesis* as the wisdom that comes from learning. He (1: 143) points out that such knowing is a very ". . . practical wisdom capable of respecting the singularity of situations as well as the nascent universality of values aimed at by human actions." If phronesis, described by Pellegrino and Thomasma (8) as *medicine's indispensable virtue*, is an outcome of operating in our patients' narratives, then narrative practitioners reap great rewards from this work. Phronesis, the ". . . capacity for moral insight, the capacity, in a given set of circumstances, to discern what moral choice or course of action is most conducive to the good of the patient", as Pellegrino and Thomasma (8: 84) describe it, is an essential element of caregiving, and a virtue that we all desire in our own physicians.

Caregivers who join with their patients in their illness narratives gain practical wisdom and are afforded the capacity to engage in broader ways of seeing and knowing. Such work often provides diagnostic or therapeutic information that may be useful in caring for patients. Information arising from illness narratives, as Greenhalgh (27: 13) points out, ". . . can be mapped to a formal disease taxonomy and coded . . ." to specific disease processes or treatments. Although traditional training in history taking and physical examination has the same aim, understanding a given patient's illness narrative may broaden the diagnostic possibilities or treatment options through the discovery of information particular to that patient's lived experience. For example, the physician in the story that opens Chapter 1 admits that additional treatment options would have been recommended more strongly if he had more fully explored the patient's narrative.

Just as many purposes are served for the caregiver in narrative work, patients also experience important benefits. Greenhalgh elaborates upon three outcomes of illness narrative exploration which accrue to patients, including the manner in which it helps the patient to understand and describe their lived experiences (27). This approach may result in a patient feeling more *heard*, and foster a more complete and understandable storytelling. Furthermore, sharing in the exploration of an illness narrative between patient and caregiver can have *illuminative value*, as the patient explores the uncertainties of illness, the ambiguities attendant on suffering and treatment, and the potential for questions to arise for which there may be no good answers. Finally, Greenhalgh describes how the *transformative value* of narrative work may lead patients to new or greater meaning as they endure the lived experience of illness. "An individual's illness narrative", she points out, "is not merely a story about the self and the illness – it is a dynamic and discursive *shaping* of the self in the face of illness." The potential to shape a different self is enabled, she argues, by the listening and trust that derive from the relationship between patient and caregiver immersed in the patient's illness story.

The healing power of illness narratives has received attention in the literature of nursing as well as that of medicine. For example, Sakalys (13) describes the greater self-knowing that arises from the exploration of illness stories. In addition, Sakalys emphasizes that healing takes place in the attachment which occurs between patient and nurse as they share in the unfolding of the patient's narrative. The power of healing through narrative practice is also documented in mental health nursing, where patients' stories often establish the platform from which all care begins. H Lea Gaydos (30: 254) describes the importance of the healing powers of narrative practice for patients with mental illness as follows:

> Patients offer their personal stories in exchange for care. They are not only seeking symptom management and a safe environment, but are also anxious to be understood and to find meaning in their self stories. Working with people to uncover deep meanings in their stories creates opportunities for healing and for hope as old self stories are rewritten and new ones are envisioned.

Gaydos (30) describes these personal stories derived from this patient–nurse relationship as the *currency of care* – a kind of health care legal tender exchanged between the patient and the nurse which buys healing, comfort, and hope for the patient, and often for the nurse as well.

Through such narrative clinical practice the caregiver receives an honoring invitation into the patient's lived experience, is invited to receive the story and join in its continued construction, and through this special invitation both sufferer and healer may find ways to be made whole.

The Landscapes of Illness Narratives

Jerome Bruner, as he explores the question of what constitutes a *good story*, writes about stories in a way that has relevance to narrative medicine work. Bruner

(7: 14) writes that all stories construct two landscapes – an *action landscape*, where the events of the story are played out, and a *consciousness landscape*, where we learn ". . . what those involved in the action know, think or feel." The action landscape comprises the events of the story, and the consciousness landscape is the landscape of the *meaning* of those events in the lives of the story's participants. These two landscapes – action and consciousness – are as essential as they are distinct. They are, as Bruner writes, ". . . the difference between Oedipus sharing Jocasta's bed before and after he learns from the messenger that she is his mother."

The relevance of Bruner's two landscapes to narratives of illness and suffering can be demonstrated by recalling the familiar story of Humpty Dumpty. Mr Dumpty's sitting, his calamitous fall, the arrival of the king's servants on horseback, and their futile attempts at Dumpty's reconstruction are the events of the story – Bruner's action landscape. The king's frustration at his relative impotence with regard to saving Mr Dumpty, the despair we imagine in the tears of Mrs Dumpty when she learns of the tragedy that has befallen her husband, the sobering acknowledgement that a life has been lost – these are the knowing, thinking, feeling parts – the consciousness landscape. We enjoy using this story as an illustration because if one operates in the consciousness landscape and contemplates Mr Dumpty's plight from the consciousness perspective of knowing, thinking, and feeling, one comes to understand the meaning of the story. This story reminds us that to be a healer requires more than all the power of the kingdom, its horses, and its men.

Attention to stories and their landscapes is relevant for all medical specialties – not just the obvious specialties of primary care. When the anesthesiologist expertly induces and maintains a woman's surgical slumber for a high-risk surgical procedure, he is operating in the action landscape. In the preoperative interview, when the patient begins to cry, worrying about who will care for her children if she fails to awaken from the anesthetic, he works in the consciousness landscape. He comes to know the meaning of the event in this patient's life, and through it the greater meaning of his own work.

Medical and nursing students meet their earliest patients in the landscapes of their stories. Over time, they are well trained to operate in their patients' action landscapes, and this is a critically important skill set – taking histories, examining patients, formulating differential diagnoses, and performing procedures. We worry little about their preparation in the action landscape. However, we worry a bit more about the extent to which their education prepares them to operate in the consciousness landscape. In fact, we worry that the rigors of clinical training, which are especially acute for physicians in residency, may teach trainees to minimize the consciousness side. However, if the patient and her suffering are why we are here, and if our work is to have meaning, we must work competently in both landscapes. In short, we must ensure that clinicians are trained to become competent narrative practitioners. How to support these skills is the subject of Chapter 6.

Narrative Medicine and Moral Imagination

Since it is never possible to fully know the lived experience of another, the ability to operate in another's narrative, both in action and in consciousness, requires the ability to imagine that other world. Such imagining in health care must occur in a moral landscape, and must be a moral pursuit. In this section we shall describe the concept of moral imagination and its application in caring for others.

Moral imagination is a term with roots in the history of modern conservatism, said to have been coined by Edmund Burke,* a British statesman and the so-called father of modern conservatism, in the eighteenth century (31). The concept of moral imagination has received broad attention in social and political discourse for generations, and has been defined and described in the literature of many disciplines and schools of thought.

According to Person (32: 2), Russell Kirk, an American political theorist, social critic, and historian, well known for having influenced twentieth-century modern conservatism, defines moral imagination as ". . . the power of knowing man, despite his weaknesses and sinful nature, as a moral being, meant for eternity. It recognizes that human beings, after all, are created in the image of God." It was, in Kirk's view, the ability to sustain a sense of *ethical truth* and abiding law even through the chaos of one's life.

Patricia Werhane (33: 34), a business ethics scholar, describes moral imagination as consisting of four different actions. On the individual level, being morally imaginative includes:

- self-reflection about oneself and one's situation
- disengaging from and becoming aware of one's situation, understanding the mental model or script dominating the situation, and envisioning possible moral conflicts or dilemmas that might arise in that context or as outcomes of the dominating scheme
- the ability to imagine new possibilities, including those that are not context-dependent and that might involve another mental model
- evaluation from a moral point of view of both the original context and its dominating mental models and the new possibilities that one has envisioned.

The study of conflict resolution has included conceptualizations of moral imagination that are also worthy of mention here. John Paul Lederach (34), well known internationally for his work in the fields of conflict transformation and peace building, believes that peace building is impossible without the four elements that comprise his view of moral imagination. He states (34: 5–6): "The first is the capacity to imagine the web of relationships. . . . This kind of

---

* Burke's best known positions on the conservative principles he espoused are contained in his writings on the French Revolution of 1789, *Reflections on the Revolution in France*, published in 1790. His views ". . . stood in defence of an increasingly embattled traditional social order" (31: 69).

imagination envisions and gives birth to relational mutuality. . . . Such vision requires humility and self-recognition." The second element is what he refers to as ". . . the discipline to sustain curiosity, a kind of imagination that lives in the untamed and mostly unexplored geographies of human interaction that lie beyond forced dualisms and polarizations." He goes on to describe that curiosity as requiring "attentiveness and continuous inquiry", and points out that "the Latin root *curiosus* formed on the term *cura* literally meaning spiritual and physical healing" (emphasis added). The third element is "an eternal belief in the creative act, the building and coaxing of imagination itself", and the fourth element is comfort with risk taking.

How moral imagination has come to be understood and applied in fields of study as varied as moral conservatism, business ethics, and peace building is instructive, since its varied definitions are woven from common threads. These commonalities include context in a moral landscape, some degree of self-knowing, active entry into an *other's* world or life experience, and hopeful reconstruction of narratives that blends the self-world with that of an *other*. Kirk's perspective has value in medical work, as health care practitioners are best positioned to serve those who seek their care if they operate from a framework in which the intrinsic *goodness* and value of those being served is understood as a given. Werhane's (33) stepwise approach, when viewed from a medical perspective, calls upon the practitioner to understand the possibilities that arise from knowing oneself, then distancing oneself from one's own contextual thinking, and finally imagining an *other* stance. From the peace-building model, we see the importance of *relational mutuality* as a means to healing.

We present these varied theoretical constructs in order to build a definition of moral imagination that is pertinent to caring for patients, and is essential for competent narrative medical practice. Similar to Werhane and Lederach, we too define moral imagination as consisting of four commitments:

1   to understand one's own values, biases, viewpoints, and brokenness as the meaningful substrate that one brings to the caregiving relationship
2   to remain open to the particularity and meaning of a patient's experience, and to attend mindfully to that particularity and meaning for the patient
3   to seek to understand the patient's lived experience, and come to operate in the narrative of that lived experience
4   to seek, within that narrative, to co-construct with the patient a new narrative aimed at healing.

Educating health professionals in ways that support these commitments is the focus of Chapter 6, and specifically we refer the reader to the section entitled "Exercising Moral Imagination and Practicing Empathy."

The Altruism Struggle

To exercise moral imagination and truly operate in the narrative of another requires the ability to place value on the welfare of others. Some degree of *other-directedness* is critical to a caring orientation that leads the caregiver into another's narrative to offer healing. The concept of altruism appears on every inventory of the so-called elements of professionalism or obligations of the professional. It is defined as the ability to place the needs of others ahead of one's own. Medical and nursing students are taught early in their training that altruism is the essence of professionalism, to the extent that professions, by definition, aim to provide service to others. Early in their development as professionals these students aspire to place the needs of their patients ahead of their own needs. Early in their education they also come to interact in the world of clinical medicine, where they encounter countless instances of physicians and other caregivers motivated by self-interest. Finally, they may begin to struggle early on with their own desires to *do well* at the same time as they are *doing good* for their patients. As a consequence, the tension between altruism and self-interest comes to weigh heavily as trainees develop their professional identities.

Kristen Renwich Monroe (35), a political psychology scholar, points out that a good deal of social science theory suggests that altruism should not exist at all, given the extensive evidence in support of self-interest as a natural human tendency. Yet, based upon her extensive study of altruists, Monroe (35: 3) concludes that ". . . altruists simply have a different way of seeing things. Where the rest of us see a stranger, altruists see a fellow human being." Her work debunks dominant theories about self-interested behavior, and allows for a way of seeing the world that is other-directed. She believes that what appears to distinguish altruistic individuals from more self-interested people (e.g. entrepreneurs) is a *world view* that causes them to see themselves as part of a *common humanity* – no different, no better, and no more or less special than anyone else (35). This world view leads altruists, according to her argument, to see everyone as deserving of well-being, and all of us as obligated to each other and to this common humanity.

The aspiration of altruism can be difficult for those whose world view is otherwise, and given the natural human tendency to act upon self-interest, young health care professionals often struggle with this expectation. That struggle is exacerbated by a purist approach to professionalism teaching that describes altruism as a moral absolute – a requirement for unequivocal selflessness in medical work. In medicine, we would argue that there really is no place for selflessness, in the truest sense of the word, because the caregiver is a critically important participant in narrative medical work. Furthermore, some degree of self-interest can be seen as appropriate. Pellegrino and Thomasma (8: 147) describe the existence of both legitimate and illegitimate self-interest, the former relating to ". . . duties that guard health, life, some measure of material well-being, the good of our families, friends . . .", and the latter concerning ". . . selfish self-interest."

The very fact that medical professionals earn a respectable living doing medical work creates a tension between altruism and self-interest that the ethicist

Albert Jonsen (36: 15) has described as ". . . the great structural paradox of medical morality." Trainees need to be exposed to the nature of this paradox and assisted in negotiating its challenges. Traditional models of medical education and medical practice promote self-interested behavior while espousing the importance of altruism. Professionals are expected to achieve an appropriate balance in this dynamic, despite the contradictions. And as Jonsen points out, the concepts of self-interest and altruism are not mutually exclusive. Those who are consistently inclined to serve others ahead of themselves will, at times, serve their own interests as well. The reverse is also true. Jonsen (36: 6) concludes that "Great moral lives are created out of the artistic harmony of both principles."

In recent years, public concerns have been expressed about the progressive deterioration of altruism as a central focus of medicine. Some of this concern has been aimed at younger physicians and health care practitioners, who are of a generation, the complaint goes, that cares more about its own needs than about those of others. Much has been written about the so-called *Me Millennium* or *Me Generation*. Lawrence Smith (37), a medical education dean, has described these generational differences more constructively. He (37: 440–41) cites a level of conflict between what he calls the *Baby Boomer* generation, members of which see ". . . professionalism predominantly in terms of hours worked and 'complete' dedication to the job", and *Generation X*, members of which value attending to their own needs and the needs of their families. This generation of young professionals appears to be more interested in achieving a healthy balance between their work lives and their personal lives, a trait that Smith acknowledges as a positive one, despite criticisms often levied by members of the Baby Boomer generation. He notes that "Baby Boomers – creating a value system based on their own life ethic – have confused work ethic with professionalism." The argument can be made that an altruistic caregiver who serves others through complete self-sacrifice compromises her most important caregiving instrument – herself. A healthier balance between work aimed at serving others and a personal life seeking personal happiness may allow for the provision of altruistic care as well as for the sustenance of a viable caregiver. It is here that the virtue of phronesis is important. Phronesis exercised in the context of caring relationships may suggest appropriate boundaries and balance for the everyday practice of the virtue of altruism. Such balance may in fact truly enhance the joy of medical work.

NARRATIVE IN THE PRACTITIONER–SELF DIMENSION

There are two people in the patient–caregiver relationship. The self-evidence of such a statement is often lost on nursing students, medical students, and residents, who spend most of their training time attempting to *do* patient care. This singular focus is reminiscent of a haunting question that I (*JZ*) was asked by a third-year medical student a number of years ago. It came up in a session with about eight or ten students who were gathered for the purpose of telling stories about the patients who most troubled them. The student was struggling with feelings that although she knew what to *do* in her patient's care (she had been taught well what to do), she didn't know how to bring herself into the relationship, to be herself, and to offer herself as a healer. She wanted to make that genuine human connection in a context other than simply *doing something* to the patient. She wanted to be there for her patient. And that was the question she asked: "Dr Zarconi, we spend all of our time *doing*. When do we get to *be?*"

This student's question highlights the importance of self-knowing and self-reflection in the development of competent caregivers. As we approach our patients' illness narratives, we bring with us complex selves, shaped by our own emotional, sociocultural, psychological, and spiritual development, our biases and convictions, our distractions within the milieu of our own stressful lived experiences, and our anxieties about our own capabilities. And if it can be agreed that the selves which we bring are, as Novack and colleagues (38) assert, our most important diagnostic and therapeutic instruments, then *calibrating* these instruments through self-awareness and reflection must be seen as critically important to the development of competent caregivers. "To engage in practice designed to enhance self-knowledge", Julia Connelly has argued (39: 145), "is a commitment to improve health care." There is consensus in the literature to support the observation that caregivers must understand themselves before they can hope to fully understand others, and must be sensitive to their own brokenness if they hope to competently manage the brokenness of their patients. More will be said about this in Chapter 6.

Sadly, for most health professions students and residents, little time is set aside for self-reflection and personal growth. The traditional emphasis on the logico-scientific dimension of medicine precludes adequate time spent in narrative ways of knowing, where trainees are more likely to examine how they are *becoming*. In a paper recommending a formal curriculum for residents in medical interviewing, Lipkin and colleagues (40: 279) highlight this problem:

> The young physician constantly encounters a wide range of patients who are facing sickness, disability, and death. The resident physician often has no special skills for facing these issues personally or with patients. So it is not surprising to find that the focus of many residents is mainly biotechnical. Asking residents in such a situation to be constantly "patient centered" without focusing time and energy on their own personal development is unrealistic and unwise.

In a study of patient case histories written by medical students over the course of their education, Flood and Soricelli (41) documented a general progression, as students became more *clinically trained*, from what we might describe as more narrative notes to more logico-scientific ones. They also noted that early in their training, students' case histories were narrative rather than analytic, contained far less clinical jargon, emphasized the patient as *co-narrator*, and often included mention of other characters in the patients' narratives. With further training, students' notes became briefer, less ponderous, and more abstract. More and more scientific terminology emerged, and both patient and physician as individuals disappeared from the descriptions. The authors see this transformation as a loss of the student's *authentic self*, as the student strives to perform in ways which are expected of them in the world of clinical medicine.

In addition to the progressive focus of medical students' case history skills toward disease management, science and technology, other aspects of their education may also impact upon their humanistic tendencies. Both medicine and nursing are professions which have been described as having the habit of *eating their young*. The education of medical students and of residents, in particular, has often been likened to the hardening experiences of military training, with inordinately long hours, high stress, great risk, and constant criticism from superiors. Audiey Kao (42), while a clinical associate at the University of Chicago Hospitals, wrote an elegant essay calling for *random acts of kindness* in the training of interns as an antidote to the exhaustion and demoralization that they experience in their residency training. "The actions we take to bolster or undermine the morale of our students set important examples", he argues (42: 14–16). How can we expect our trainees to give empathy when they scarcely receive any themselves during their training? How can we emphasize the importance of understanding the lived experience of sufferers when we ignore the suffering of our students and residents?

In addition, many nurses and physicians find themselves longing for opportunities to reignite a sense of calling in their work. Advances in the science and technology of medicine, pressures toward productivity, and the increasing business and profit objectives of medicine allow less and less opportunity for reflection by practitioners on the meaning of their work, and on the joys of serving the suffering. Satisfaction with medical careers may decline as a result. In their 2004 survey of physicians, Merritt, Hawkins & Associates (43) reported declining satisfaction among physicians between 2000 and 2004. Interestingly, in both survey years approximately 60% of the physicians who were surveyed identified patient relationships as their *single greatest source of professional satisfaction*. Growing numbers of physicians and, we suspect, also nurses long to recapture their interest and commitment to enter the lives and stories of their patients, and to return to their work there as healers, as the most important responsibility that they fulfill.

Witness, for example, the emergence of the Finding Meaning in Medicine (FMM) movement as evidence of growing physician dysphoria. Since 2000, Rachel Naomi Remen's Institute for the Study of Health and Illness (ISHI) has been inviting physicians from all over the country to learn to conduct, in their own communities, Finding Meaning in Medicine programs aimed at physicians who long to *reclaim the heart and soul of medicine* in their work. This program has been extremely successful in its efforts to spawn FMM meetings in the homes of physicians all over the USA, a number that continues to grow, presumably in proportion to the extent to which physicians are struggling to sustain a sense of their calling to medicine. Remen's website invitation into the FMM program (44) calls to physicians who are suffering the strains of contemporary medical practice, and asks physicians to consider whether they still experience joy in medicine, desire a community of like-minded physicians motivated by caring and service, and hope to rekindle the sense of meaning in their work. I (JZ) had an opportunity to attend an FMM conference, and found it to be one of the most powerful experiences of my career. It was a poignant reminder of why I pursued a life of service in medicine, and it offered hope of rekindling the joy of medical work through greater focus on the illness narratives of my patients.

While Jennifer Bau was a student at Pennsylvania State University College of Medicine, she encountered a self-portrait painted by a woman who had undergone mastectomy for breast cancer. She was so moved by this painting that she wrote a poem entitled *Sag*, as a description of the medical world from which this patient's experiences arose, and of her own sagging spirit. Her poem (45: 19–20) opens with dictionary definitions of the word "sag", including the concept of drooping or settling as a result of weight or pressure as well as that of losing "strength, firmness, or resilience." Jennifer's poem captures many of the dimensions of what Kao (42) would describe as the demoralizing experiences of training, as a busy student is forced to turn away from the human dimension of suffering with cancer and losing a breast to ". . . understanding the importance/ Of axillary and cutaneous lymph nodes . . .". In a quiet moment in the library, the student ponders the painting, eyelids sagging:

> And she murmurs,
>> Hope all those healing snakes are standard
>> When my white coat
>> Is long enough for respect
>> Because it sure would be nice
>> To not have to do everything
>> All by myself.

The poem describes an emerging sense of loneliness in the training of the medical student, and a sagging spirit. It concludes quite poignantly as the patient makes a strenuous attempt to remind the highly stressed caregivers what is most important in their work:

> Cries out to the jaded journeyers
>> We don't want everything you have
>> And you don't have to be everything to us
>> Just make sure that we're surrounded
>> By more hands
>> Than we can hold.

The connection between patient and caregiver, in Bau's imagining, is the essential ingredient for healing. The student's engagement in the imaginative writing of poetry, we believe, is an attempt to sustain her authentic self as healer.

Self-Awareness, Reflective Learning, and Practice

The ability to know and sustain one's authentic self is critically important in the development of the caregiver. Yet most of traditional caregiver training turns attention away from the self toward the work of diagnosing and treating disease. Furthermore, the premedical focus of the typical nursing and medical student is generally science based, and is thus less likely to have fostered extensive self-reflection, self-exploration and self-knowing than would be found in the humanities and social sciences. "Many learners in the health professions", argue Jane Westberg and Hilliard Jason (46: 2), ". . . live in cultures in which 'doing' and 'being productive' are highly valued, and quiet reflection is neglected or devalued." The importance of a caregiver's awareness of self is emphasized by Sharon Dobie, family physician and educator, who writes (47: 424):

> Self-awareness is what differentiates us from others, providing a key to the possibility of actually knowing another while giving us the matrix for healthy boundaries in the relationships we form. Our relationships with patients provide us with many opportunities to learn about ourselves. Most of us know this, even if we do not speak about it. Educators now face the task to intentionally teach this insight and to expect that learners will actively work on self-awareness at the same time that they learn and practice their other medical skills.

Thus efforts to foster self-reflection in the training of caregivers become as important as those aimed at cognitive and skills training. Westberg and Jason (46: 2–10) describe the importance of balancing the classroom and clinical experiential lessons with activities aimed at self-reflective skills, and cite a number of important reasons for such an approach, which can be summarized as follows:

Reasons for Fostering Self-Reflection

1 Too many health-profession learners do not have well-developed reflection skills.
2 The skills of reflection, including self assessment, can be learned.
3 Reflection enables learners to identify and build on their existing knowledge.
4 Reflection can enable learners to identify deficits in their knowledge and errors in their thinking.
5 Reflection can enable learners to generalize from particular experiences and apply this new knowledge in later situations.
6 Reflection can help learners to integrate new understanding.

7 With reflection, including self-assessment, learning can be accelerated.

8 Reflection can enable learners to identify unexamined assumptions and biases that can interfere with learning and patient care.

9 Reflection can enable learners to be in touch with their feelings so that they can take care of themselves and provide compassionate and comprehensive care.

10 Learners are likely to feel more ownership of insights that emerge from their own discoveries.

11 Learners can feel more self-respect and confidence if they identify their deficiencies and strengths.

12 Learners' reflections can focus us [educators] more accurately on what they need.

13 Inviting learners' reflections can help us to foster collaborative relationships with them.

14 To be competent and to continue learning throughout their careers, health professionals need to be reflective practitioners.

15 Reflective practitioners are likely to provide better patient care.

16 Health professionals who are not reflective, self-directed, self-critical learners can become incompetent, and even dangerous.

We believe that most students pursue careers in nursing and medicine out of a desire to help people in need. It is clear that in order to sustain such motivations, students, guided by well-meaning faculty, must be given ample opportunity to nurture their authentic selves throughout their training in ways that strengthen rather than diminish their narrative and humanistic commitments. Caregivers would do well to seek ways throughout their careers to sustain and nurture their caring selves through the practice of self-reflective work aimed at their humanistic commitments. Again, more will be said about this in Chapter 6.

Reflective learning and practice are critically important in the development of narrative practitioners. Gillie Bolton (48: xiii), a senior research fellow at King's College London, defines reflective practice as ". . . generously giving time, enthusiasm and insight into your experience, knowledge and feelings, and – perhaps most vitally – warmth." She describes this focus on the self as a process of *minding the gap* (48: xv):

> Bank Underground Station, London, is built on a curve, leaving a potentially dangerous gap between platform and carriage to trap the unwary. The loud-speaker voice instructs passengers to *'Mind the gap'* – the boundary between train and platform. *Gap* can be used as an image for other boundaries in our lives, such as between professional me and parent me. We spend our lives minding gaps to protect ourselves from being hit by trains, eaten by bears (Milne, 1924) [49] or falling into uncomfortable situations where we do not know the answers. Awareness of such gaps can lead to deep, thorough self-

questioning. At such moments of openness, understanding can flash: 'aha' moments of 'oh, I see!', epiphanies of allowing myself to stop thinking, stop carefully being myself, and allow other possibilities to present themselves. At these times and places professionals are open to querying, or potentially querying, situations, knowledge, feeling and understandings. Such deeply reflective questions are bridges which cross moral gulfs.

Educational experiences specifically directed at development of self-awareness in students and residents may serve as an antidote to traditional medical enculturation or socialization. When a new curriculum was adopted at our medical school, the Northeastern Ohio Universities College of Medicine (NEOUCOM), faculty sought to create spaces apart from the basic sciences for first- and second-year students to reflect on their own values and beliefs as they interacted with biomedicine and medical education. The focus in these "Reflections on Doctoring" sessions has been on their lives here and now, rather than abstract discussions of compassion or remote cases in bioethics before they have ever seen patients. In addition to the assignment of short readings – often short stories, autobiographical essays, or poetry – students are required to write short self-reflective essays on the topics under discussion. These have included sexual identity, substance abuse and impairment, cheating, or dissection of their cadaver. The attempt has been to gather faculty who have a calling to teach, not to preach, who model self-reflection and vulnerability, and who have a strong interest in promoting humanism in medicine.

In addition, during several core clerkship rotations in their third year, students engage in reflective writing exercises related to patient experiences which have troubled them, or their critical experiences with the so-called hidden curriculum. These opportunities for critical self-reflection in safe spaces with trusted faculty are seen by internist and educator William Branch (50) as necessary for the moral development of medical students. Citing the analysis of moral development by the psychologist Kohlberg, Branch suggests that medical students experience delays, or even regression, in their moral development in clinical environments where they experience conflict between doing what they believe to be right for their patients, and following the conventions demonstrated by their superiors in order to *fit in* as members of the health care team. Fearing reprisals that could negatively impact on their academic advancement, it is conceivable that when they experience such conflict, students subjugate their own moral impulses and thus come to operate in a state of *sustained adolescence* with regard to their moral development. It becomes critical that we ensure our students' participation in self-reflective work through these important rites of passage, and that we continue to develop and sustain a community of faculty who are capable of consistently supporting and mentoring these students along the way.

At the resident level, we recently implemented a year-long narrative medicine curriculum within the family medicine residency program at our health system. The program is a mixture of didactic and interactive work, including exposure to medical readers' theater, imaginative literature, poetry, art, and film. Although the course is directed at second-year residents, all residents, faculty, and staff are invited. Participants engage in reflective writing and sharing throughout the course. After the first year, participants commented that these reflective activities were quite meaningful – indeed helpful – to them. Some observed that self-reflective work was not something in which they would otherwise have been engaged during the rigors of their residency training, and they appreciated these opportunities.

Novack and colleagues (38: 502–5) propose a curricular approach to enhancing physician self-development and personal awareness that they define as "... insight into how one's life experiences and emotional make-up affect one's interactions with patients, families, and other professionals." The core topics of their curriculum, it seems to us, bear applicability to the development of self in other health care professions as well, and are reproduced below:

A Core Curriculum for Physician Personal Awareness

Physician's beliefs and attitudes
Core beliefs/personal philosophy
Family-of-origin influences
Gender issues
Sociocultural influences

Physician's feelings and emotional responses concerning patient care
Love, caring, attraction, and boundary setting
Conflict/anger

Challenging clinical situations
"Difficult" patients
Caring for dying patients
Medical mistakes

Physician self-care
Balancing personal and professional lives
Preventing and managing stress/burnout/impairment

Whatever the curriculum or educational approach, clearly the caregiver–self must be nourished and provided with an opportunity for continued growth and development. The caregivers' own narratives and their authentic selves are important to the healing work that they hope to bring to the relationships which they have with their patients. As educators, we are obligated to ensure that our students' and residents' educational experiences are structured so as to sustain and nurture their caring selves in very conscious ways. For a health professional to competently operate in the narrative of a patient, she must have mastered the caregiver–self domain through conscious exploration, questioning, evaluation, and growth of the self in ways aimed at becoming a healer. Such self-knowing is akin to what Maxine Greene describes as *wide-awakeness*, and as she points out (51: 12), "Wide-awakeness leads to epiphanies."

FURTHER ACTIVITIES

1 Readers who are interested in exploring Jerome Bruner's descriptions of the elements of story in more detail are encouraged to read the following: Bruner J. *Actual Minds, Possible Worlds*. Cambridge, MA: Harvard University Press; 1986.

2 Readers who are interested in the work of Rachel Naomi Remen in helping practitioners to reclaim a sense of meaning in their work are encouraged to visit Remen's website: http://meaninginmedicine.org.

REFERENCES

1 Kearney R. *On Stories*. New York: Routledge; 2002.

2 Fredriksson L, Eriksson K. The patient's narrative of suffering: a path to health? *Scand J Caring Sci*. 2001; **15**: 3–11.

3 Charon R. Narrative of human plight: a conversation with Jerome Bruner. In: Charon R, Montello M, editors. *Stories Matter: the role of narrative in medical ethics*. New York: Routledge; 2002. pp. 3–9.

4 Stevens W. *The Collected Poems of Wallace Stevens*. New York: Vintage; 1990.

5 Rilke RM. *Rainer Maria Rilke: selected poems*. New York: Routledge; 1986.

6 Charon R. Narrative medicine: a model for empathy, reflection, profession, and trust. *JAMA*. 2001; **286:** 1897–902.

7 Bruner J. *Actual Minds, Possible Worlds*. Cambridge, MA: Harvard University Press; 1986.

8 Pellegrino ED, Thomasma DC. *The Virtues in Medical Practice*. New York: Oxford University Press; 1993.

9 Donovan GK. The physician–patient relationship. In: Thomasma DC, Kissell JL, editors. *The Health Care Professional as Friend and Healer: building on the work of Edmund D Pellegrino*. Washington, DC: Georgetown University Press; 2000. pp. 13–23.

10 Cassell EJ. *The Nature of Suffering and the Goals of Medicine*. New York: Oxford University Press; 1991.

11 Davis FD. Friendship as an ideal for the patient–physician relationship: a critique and an alternative. In: Thomasma DC, Kissell JL, editors. *The Health Care Professional as Friend and Healer: building on the work of Edmund D Pellegrino*. Washington, DC: Georgetown University Press; 2000. pp. 24–34.

12 Frank AW. *The Wounded Storyteller*. Chicago, IL: University of Chicago Press; 1995.

13 Sakalys JA. Restoring the patient's voice: the therapeutics of illness narratives. *J Holist Nurs*. 2003; **21:** 228–41.

14 Coles R. *The Call of Stories*. Boston, MA: Houghton Mifflin; 1989.

15 Whitehead AN. *Science and the Modern World*. San Francisco, CA: Collins Fontana; 1975.

16 Brody H. *The Healer's Power*. New Haven, CT: Yale University Press; 1992.

17 Starr P. *The Social Transformation of American Medicine: the rise of a sovereign profession and the making of a vast industry*. New York: Basic Books; 1982.

18 Friedson E. *Profession of Medicine: a study of the sociology of applied knowledge*. Chicago, IL: University of Chicago Press; 1988.

19 Montgomery K. *How Doctors Think: clinical judgment and the practice of medicine*. Oxford: Oxford University Press; 2006.

20 Rimmon-Kenan S. The story of "I": illness and narrative identity. *Narrative*. 2002; 10: 9–27.

21 Roter DL, Hall JA. *Doctors Talking with Patients/Patients Talking with Doctors: improving communication in medical visits*. 2nd ed. Westport, CT: Praeger; 2006.

22 Szasz TS, Hollender MH. The basic models of the doctor–patient relationship. *Arch Intern Med*. 1956; 97: 585–92.

23 Emanuel EJ, Emanuel LL. Four models of the physician–patient relationship. *JAMA*. 1992; 267: 2221–6.

24 Yedidia MJ. Transforming doctor–patient relationships to promote patient-centered care: lessons from palliative care. *J Pain Symptom Manage*. 2007; 33: 40–57.

25 McArthur JH, Moore FD. The two cultures and the health care revolution. *JAMA*. 1997; 277: 985–9.

26 Brody H. *Stories of Sickness*. New York: Oxford University Press; 2003.

27 Greenhalgh T. *What Seems to be the Trouble? Stories in illness and healthcare*. Oxford: Radcliffe Publishing; 2006.

28 Charon R. *Narrative Medicine: honoring the stories of illness*. New York: Oxford University Press; 2006.

29 Aull F. Telling and listening: constraints and opportunities. *Narrative*. 2005; 13: 281–93.

30 Gaydos, HL. Understanding personal narratives: an approach to practice. *J Adv Nurs*. 1998; 49: 254–9.

31 Heywood A. *Political Ideologies: an introduction*. New York: Palgrave Macmillan; 2003.

32 Person JE. *The achievement of Russell Kirk. (Russell Kirk and the Age of Ideology)* (book review); www.encyclopedia.com

33 Werhane PH. Moral imagination and systems thinking. *J Bus Ethics*. 2002; 38: 33–42.

34 Lederach JP. *The moral imagination: the art and soul of building peace*. In: Association of Conflict Resolution 2004 Annual Conference Keynote Presentation; www.acrnet. org/conferences/ac04/lederachspeech.htm

35 Monroe KR. *The Heart of Altruism: perception of a common humanity*. Princeton, NJ: Princeton University Press; 1996.

36 Jonsen AR. *The New Medicine and the Old Ethics*. Cambridge, MA: Harvard University Press; 1990.

37 Smith LG. Medical professionalism and the generation gap. *Am J Med*. 2005; 118: 439–42.

38 Novack DH, Suchman AL, Clark W *et al*. for the Working Group on Promoting Physician Personal Awareness, American Academy on Physician and Patient.

Calibrating the physician: personal awareness and effective patient care. *JAMA.* 1997; **278:** 502–9.

39 Connelly JE. In the absence of narrative. In: Charon R, Montello M, editors. *Stories Matter: the role of narrative in medical ethics.* New York: Routledge; 2002. pp. 138–46.

40 Lipkin M, Quill TE, Napodano RJ. The medical interview: a core curriculum for residencies in internal medicine. *Ann Intern Med.* 1984; **100:** 277–84.

41 Flood DH, Soricelli RL. Development of the physician's narrative voice in the medical case history. *Lit Med.* 1992; **11:** 64–83.

42 Kao A. Random acts of kindness: sustaining the morale and morals of professionalism. In: *Professing Medicine, Commemorative Issue of Virtual Mentor* (American Medical Association's online ethics journal); www.virtualmentor.org

43 Merritt, Hawkins and Associates. *2004 Survey of Physicians 50 to 65 Years Old*; http://merritthawkins.com/compensation_surveys.cfm

44 Remen RN; http://meaninginmedicine.org

45 Bau J. Sag. In: *Professing Medicine, Commemorative Issue of Virtual Mentor* (American Medical Association's online ethics journal); www.virtualmentor.org

46 Westberg J, Jason H. *Fostering Reflection and Providing Feedback.* New York: Springer; 2001.

47 Dobie S. Viewpoint: reflections on a well-travelled path: self-awareness, mindful practice, and relationship-centered care as foundations for medical education. *Acad Med.* 2007; **82:** 422–7.

48 Bolton G. *Reflective Practice: writing and professional development.* 2nd ed. London: Sage; 2001.

49 Milne AA. *The World of Christopher Robin (When We Were Very Young).* London: Methuen; 1924.

50 Branch WT. Supporting the moral development of medical students. *J Gen Intern Med.* 2000; **15:** 503–8.

51 Greene M. Towards wide-awakeness: humanities in the lives of professionals. In: Wear D, Kohn M, Stocker S, editors. *Literature and medicine: a claim for a discipline.* McLean, VA: Society for Health and Human Values; 1987. pp. 3–15.

CHAPTER 5

Narrative Contexts of Profession and Community

> All human communities rely on healers to elaborate conceptions of health and wholeness, and apply their expertise for the benefit of individuals and societies.
>
> **Daniel George, Iahn Gonsenhauser,**
> **and Peter Whitehouse (1: 63)**

> ... narrativists like to emphasize the crucial role that stories play in socializing people into accepted ways of acting, thinking, and perceiving, in fostering group cohesion, and in perpetuating communal traditions. . . . Narratives, then, are what constitute community.
>
> **Lewis P Hinchman and Sandra K Hinchman (2: 235)**

KEY IDEAS

- The narrative of the profession of medicine has been described as having turned, over time, from one that described the provision of valuable service to society toward one characterized by more self-interested and commercial motivations among its members.

- Health professional trainees experience significant contradictions between what they are taught in the classroom regarding their professional obligations and what they see enacted by professionals in the *real world* of clinical medicine. How they respond to these contradictions critically influences the development of their professional identities.

- Contemporary narratives of professionalism have called for greater emphasis in health professional education on narrative competence, self-awareness, reflective practice, and commitments to community service and public health.

- Recommendations for health professional educators to promote these contemporary narratives of professionalism are presented.

- The newest generation of health professionals appears to be characterized by greater commitments to balance between their personal and professional lives, and is inclined toward obligations set internally rather than by external institutions and social structures. Curricula and training environments aimed at this generation of young professionals must be constructed with attention to these attributes.

- If medicine is to truly function as a community, it must continue to renew its narratives in the light of contemporary health care concerns, address the forces which serve to divide its members, re-examine its commitments to serve the suffering and the public, and ensure the training of its next generation of members.

- The broader understanding of suffering and health that arises from narrative medical practice can contribute to healthier communities.

INTRODUCTION

In Chapter 4 we described the importance of narrative in both the patient–practitioner and the practitioner–self relationship. As we now turn to consider narrative within the domains of profession and community, we intend to reframe the scholarly work on these topics from a narrative stance. While all professions have evolved with unique storylines that could be examined, we focus on the profession of medicine, and specifically physicians, since this literature is replete with storylines of its evolution as a profession.*

Various disciplines, including the fields of sociology, philosophy and ethics,

---

* Rich descriptions of the development of medicine as profession exist in the literatures of sociology, ethics, and medicine itself, and we refer the reader in particular to the works of Creuss *et al.* (3, 4), and Hafferty (5) for detailed discussions of this literature.

education, and medicine, take different approaches in their depictions and analyses of the concept of profession – they construct different stories to situate profession from the particular perspectives of their disciplines. One can view these perspectives as continual re-emplotments of storylines, bound in particular times and social contexts. These storylines are generally constructed in the service of persuasion – intended to persuade people bound within a given period or context who are trying to make sense of the core values of profession, who are attempting to live and work within these core values, and who hope to transmit these core values to subsequent generations within the profession. The storylines are constructed in the service of persuasion of those outside the profession as well. How a society comes to view the profession, what it expects, and what the profession gives in return, are all fundamentally influenced by the stories that profession constructs. These narratives, when viewed over time, have implications for how the work of a profession is enacted, how a profession becomes situated within broader sociocultural constructs, and how a profession's core values are sustained and passed on to future members.

It is in this context that we intend to describe narrative concepts within the practitioner–profession and practitioner–community domains. We begin with a discussion of the medical profession's narrative as it has evolved to the present. We then describe the implications of that narrative for future generations of the profession in the context of medical education. Finally, we assess medicine's storyline as it relates to the concept of community, attempting to depict how a community narrative might offer hope for a profession's power to heal.

NARRATIVE IN THE PRACTITIONER–PROFESSION DIMENSION
The Narrative of Medicine as Profession

The earliest narratives of the concept of profession date back to the early twentieth century. Most scholars credit Justice Louis Brandeis (6) with having formulated the earliest definition of profession. Brandeis wrote that professions are characterized by three key features – specialized knowledge training, work in service to others, and emphasis on non-monetary rewards. This conceptualization evolved considerably in the ensuing decades, and numerous observers have delineated additional characteristics of profession. Creuss and Creuss (4) present a summary of what we would agree are the important additional elements of profession. They include the following (4: 944):

- knowledge and skills controlled exclusively by its members
- work controlled and organized by independent associations
- licensing and authority-granting power
- expectation of influencing public awareness and policy
- control over admission to and education for the profession
- control over terms and conditions of practice
- code of ethics

- autonomy in the work of the profession
- expectation of public service
- higher standards of behavior
- expectation of morality.

There appears to be agreement in the literature that the essence of a profession is its specialized knowledge and skills and the application of these in service to others. In this storyline, the autonomy granted the profession comes in return for the profession's commitment to that service ethic and the vow that its members take to place the needs of others ahead of their own needs. The social contract, as it has been described, that derives from this narrative will be further discussed later in this chapter.

The early twentieth-century literature on professions, even into the 1950s and early 1960s, is generally a storyline of beneficence, descriptive of the benefits of professions as useful in organizing work, inclined toward service, and helpful in providing stability in a society whose institutions are being diminished by industrial progress. This storyline began to shift in the 1960s as the profession of medicine continued to expand its sociocultural and organizational powers in ways that demonstrated progressively greater self-interest among its members and the profession as a whole. A re-emplotment of this narrative to a more critical stance toward the profession of medicine arose from the writings of Eliot Friedson (7) in the late 1960s and early 1970s. He described the *impurity* of professional authority, and developed his *professional dominance theory*. Friedson criticized organized medicine's autonomy, noting that this autonomy resulted from persuading the public of medicine's trustworthiness. He further contended that the story of medicine was shifting toward inordinate self-interest and insufficient self-regulation, and moving away from its central ethic of service.

Subsequent critics of medicine as a profession began to depict medicine's narratives as characterized by *deprofessionalization* (8), *proletarianization* (9), and *corporatization* (10). These storylines describe a shift toward profit motivation and medicine as business. Such a shift has exacerbated the tension between altruism and self-interest described previously. McArthur and Moore (11) have described these two cultures of service provision as professional and commercial – the former focused on patient welfare, and the latter motivated by profit. They further specify the many hazards that arise when medicine's focus becomes the achievement of an excess of revenue over expense, rather than serving the suffering. They warn, for example, of the potential growth of the population that is unable to afford services, the exclusion of high-risk patients from available services, undue burden on public service providers, downgrading of the qualifications of health care providers, growth of entrepreneurship among clinicians and researchers, and neglect of the obligations to support teaching and research in medicine, as some of these commercial culture hazards.

Contemporary Narratives of Professionalism

Contemporary narratives of medicine demonstrate the manner in which medicine has moved away from its primary service ethic. While patients often celebrate their physicians' knowledge and technical skills, increasingly they lament that they feel unheard and/or uncared for by those physicians. Greater public attention has been focused on physicians' relationships with industry – not least of which is the pharmaceutical industry – including physicians' equity participation across a broad range of the health care services industry. Research scandals have become more public if not more commonplace. Stimulated perhaps by narratives found in the Institute of Medicine reports (12, 13), medical errors and patient safety issues have become central foci for health care. Even physicians worry, when they experience illness or injury and become patients themselves, that their doctors and health care institutions will not serve them appropriately. Gibbs and Bower (14) note that physicians as patients often know too much, having witnessed the distortions of the health care system that arise from litigation concerns, insurance industry influences, business competition, growing bureaucracy, and increasingly risk-laden technologies.

Into this narrative milieu arrives the next generation of physicians – medical students and residents. They arrive in the clinical arena having spent time in classrooms, small group discussions, and other curriculum activities in which they have been exposed to the stories of professionalism. These stories portray the profession's history and the commitments that they are expected to be making. Through these narrative portraits, students and residents come to understand *the rules and requirements* of the profession. Much of this comes to them from faculty whom Castellani and Hafferty (15) describe as *nostalgic professionals*, and the *ruling class* of medicine. This teaching narrative, what one of our students characterized as *preaching from the pulpit of professionalism*, is meant to persuade students toward a life of service in medicine. As Castellani and Hafferty (15: 12) point out, this group of nostalgic professionals:

> . . . advocates (attempts to re-establish) a "professionalism of old" for which they long – a professionalism that is grounded in autonomy and dominance and that houses an immense disdain for commercialism. It is within this narrative that commercialism is most unilaterally cast as the antithesis and enemy of "medical professionalism." Their solution is to re-establish professional dominance over it. In this way, nostalgic professionalism is conventional, mainstream medical professionalism, as it has been idealized by organized medicine and the social services for the past hundred years (e.g. Starr, 1982).

Distressingly, however, when medical students don their white coats and enter the world of clinical medicine alongside residents and other professionals, they immediately experience contradictions of what they have learned. Students find themselves immersed in what Thomas Inui (16) has described as a clear gap between what professionals espouse as virtuous practice and what those professionals actually do in their day-to-day work. They witness attitudes and behaviors that demonstrate professionalism counter-narratives. They learn *how it really is* in medicine, as they are introduced to physicians who have financial relationships with pharmaceutical companies, or who own and operate laboratory or diagnostic facilities to which they refer their patients. They see physicians who behave inappropriately or demonstrate incompetence, often without consequences. They are mistreated. In the 2006 American Association of Medical Colleges (AAMC) Medical School Graduation Questionnaire (17), 12% of the more than 11,000 medical student respondents acknowledged such mistreatment. Included are instances of public humiliation (sometimes frequent), as well as gender and ethnic discrimination. Despite what they have been taught about compassion and respect, they witness examples of patients and families being treated inappropriately. They witness derogatory humor directed at patients, and in fact are expected to join in these behaviors as fully integrated team members (18). They often remain silent regarding these witnessed transgressions, mostly out of fear of reprisal (17), and many students describe a sense of powerlessness in reporting, believing little if anything will be done in response to such complaints. These storylines teach a view of medicine as a profession in which physicians advance their own positions, see patients in negative ways, and disregard the obligations that the students learned about in more *nostalgic* lessons on professionalism. In the face of these counter-narratives, prior classroom lessons on professionalism begin to fall flat. As Daniel George and colleagues note (1: 63), ". . . noble abstractions are uttered, commendable pronouncements are made, but because there is no sustained attempt to filter them through the cultural realities students face, they are not reinforced and are instead perceived as ivory-tower propaganda", as narratives of falsehood and deceit. It should come as no surprise then that the cynicism which begins to take hold of these developing professionals results in part from their experiences with these contradictions. As Inui points out (16: 16), ". . . students learn that medicine *is* a profession in which you say one thing and do another, a profession of cynics."

In recent decades, medical education institutions have attempted to shift the dominant narrative by focusing more attention on humanistic approaches, relationship-centered models of care, communication skills training, and the like, yet the health care system does not appear to have been influenced in more positive directions. Not surprisingly, in recent years numerous constituencies within organized medicine have been attempting to re-narrate professionalism through major reforms. The American Board of Internal Medicine developed its *Project Professionalism*, and then in cooperation with the American College of Physicians–American Society of Internal Medicine and the European Federation of Internal Medicine, it developed the *Medical Professionalism Project* of 2002, from which came the *Charter on Medical Professionalism*, which was published in two major medical journals (19, 20). The American Association of Medical Colleges (AAMC) developed a major initiative focused on professionalism education, as did the Accreditation Council for Graduate Medical Education (ACGME), which identified professionalism as one of its six core competencies. Both organizations have implemented expectations for medical schools and graduate medical education programs, respectively, to incorporate professionalism teaching (AAMC) and to measure professionalism competency outcomes (ACGME). Professionalism is now one of the hottest topics in organized medicine and medical education – a narrative which urges renewal of early traditions and obligations. As Coulehan writes, professionalism is now ". . . springing like kudzu from every nook and cranny of medical education" (21: 104).

This contemporary professionalism fervor, although laudable and offering hope of a return by medicine to its ideals and service ethic, is not without its detractors. Chief among them may be our medical students, who have begun to tire of what many now call the *P word*. At our institution (Northeastern Ohio Universities College of Medicine), and as we have heard from colleagues around the country at many other medical schools, no word causes more medical students' eyes to roll upward, or causes more students to either stop listening or even become angry or frustrated with us, as the word *professionalism*. Students have begun to construct a resistive counter-narrative in response, perhaps, to misinterpretations of professionalism by educators. We believe that too many well-meaning educators have confused professionalism conversations with conversations about rules of common decency, civil behavior, and issues related to the *Golden Rule*. When our students come late to class, we haul out our professionalism sticks. When they wear open-toed sandals, flash their tattoos, talk to each other during class, fail to turn off their cell phones, or fail to turn in their course evaluation forms, we haul out our professionalism sticks. Students get so tired of being rebuked in the name of professionalism that their minds close at the mere mention of the word. Although the achievement of a professional ethic is made more difficult without the consistent incorporation of decency in behavior, educators must push for clearer narrative distinctions between how we expect our students to behave (without relating that to professionalism), and the commitments we want our students to reflect on, aspire to, and profess as physicians. It is important to construct narratives of professionalism that help our students to understand that *how they act* is important, and that breeches in appropriate behavior have consequences that might include disciplinary measures. We must nurture our students' own exploration of what they hope to bring to their work as physicians, what they intend to commit to, and what they will profess, and only call that professionalism. We should refer to what they do and how they act in terms of common decency, and speak of who they are becoming as related to professionalism.

This narrative confusion over the concept of professionalism is further complicated by the gradual and continuous evolution of its emplotment over time as seen in the literature. Too often, professionalism is portrayed as a static concept despite its ever changing meanings in medical education and in health care systems. Sharon Johnston (22: 186) points out that:

> ... it can be viewed as a dynamic framework derived from the interaction of many forces, such as the tradition of healing, social change, rising medical challenges, and scientific advances, as well as the interests of members and subgroups within and outside the profession.

The challenges of professionalism and its profound obligations must be part of the educational push, and trainees and members of the profession must be encouraged to reflect on what these challenges mean in the lived experience of contemporary medical work. Julia Connelly (23) expresses concern that one of professionalism's tenets – to place patients' interests ahead of one's own – is voiced without explanations as to what it requires. As mentioned in Chapter 4, aspiring professionals often struggle mightily with the difficulties associated with suppression of self-interest to extremes that may ultimately diminish the professional power of the self. Connelly goes on to levy further criticisms of the contemporary professionalism push, including the continued tendency to deny limitations, the persistent emphasis on caregivers developing emotional detachment, the logico-scientific focus of professionalism, the continued call for serving society while the number of people without access to care continues to grow, and the continued evidence of self-interested behavior on the part of the medical profession. Connelly argues that the essential narrative of professionalism should be refocused as obligations of the entire profession in contrast to individual responsibility. She posits (23: 182):

> ... if one of the central aims of medical professionalism that "demands placing the interests of the patients above those of the physician" is revised to apply to the profession as a whole, the revised statement might read: an obligation to put the interests of the public (that pertain to health and well-being) before the interests of the medical profession. This aim alone clarifies the role and obligation of medical societies to support the greater good rather than their turf and membership. It pushes medical organizations toward supporting some type of universal health insurance, and it calls for serious reflection and decision making regarding medicine's involvement with and dependence on pharmaceutical companies.

It is conceivable that much of what may thwart the professional development of medical students and young physicians is an oppressive sense of being individually unable to fully and conscientiously live up to professionalism's obligations so stated. A narrative of a *collective* living up may strengthen medicine's functioning as a community, and enhance the profession's chances of restoring the primacy of its patient focus.

Fred Hafferty (24) has reviewed the stories of professionalism within the narrative descriptions of sociology, medicine, and education, and his review highlights the changing nature of professionalism's meanings and implications – its narrative. He concludes his review by presenting the features of professionalism from what he terms a *new professionalism* narrative, from the US as well as the UK literature. He observes that more contemporary medical literature on professionalism has provided a complex storyline that advocates for mindfulness, the importance of personal reflection and *reflexiveness*, professional identity development, and self-evaluation as critical elements of professionalism. He (24) goes on to describe the contemporary sociological literature on professionalism as having three major orientations, key features of which include:

- *responsive professionalism,* which requires reflection, demands a responsiveness to lay persons and the community, and clearly references altruism
- *civic professionalism,* which is built upon civic engagement and a mutuality of obligation, has clear moral and ethical dimensions, and is enacted by self-aware practitioners
- *democratic professionalism,* recognizing fairness and social justice as central ethics, with a focus on advocacy for patients, clear emphasis on responsibility for the health of populations and improved health outcomes, and characterized by evidence-based practice.

These descriptions are useful as educators ponder the scope and nature of the professionalism education that must be directed toward the next generation of health professionals. It appears that an emerging understanding of professionalism over time has built toward a strong focus on re-engaging with communities in a model of professionalism characterized by patient-centeredness. Such sociological storylines, when superimposed upon medical narratives that emphasize self-reflective practice as a critical element of professionalism, begin to construct a contemporary narrative of professionalism which will probably require new forms of training and role modeling. Emphasis in such training on the powerful narratives that unfold in the patient–practitioner, practitioner–self, practitioner–profession, and practitioner–community domains, and on how caring and healing arise from such narratives, seems likely to support the development of a profession with greater abilities to fulfill its contract with society.

Creuss and colleagues (3) argue that this is a time of great opportunity for the profession to regain its status of trust and reaffirm its commitments to service. They recommend broader education of physicians and trainees regarding the history described above and the obligations of professionalism. In addition, they encourage a recommitment to self-regulation and policy within the profession, further expansion of knowledge and research, and a refocusing on community health.

Members of the medical profession are more likely to pursue such a path of renewal and healing, we would argue, if they are able to experience greater meaning in their work, and deeper understanding of its privilege as well as its obligations. In addition, renewal is more likely to be achieved if these efforts are pursued collectively across the profession rather than by individuals. Greater experiences in the narratives of our patients, in each other's narratives, and in the narratives of the profession are likely to facilitate such renewal. Individual physicians can begin by refocusing on the meaning of profession in their own particular narratives, and by greater sharing of these narratives among colleagues. Organized medicine must seek ways to reunite its members, and lead an expansive education and recommitment endeavor across the medical community, including trainees. Charon's (25) concepts of *attention*, *representation*, and *affiliation*, consciously and competently applied, could prove invaluable to such pursuits, and just may reconnect the profession with the people and communities whom it hopes to serve in more meaningful ways.

Implications for Medical Education

Sharon Johnston (22) has stressed that professionalism is influenced by social change, stating that subsequent generations of physicians renegotiate the moral underpinnings of professionalism in such a way that they are consistent with the historically framed values of society. These actions are transacted through narrative means. It behoves us as educators to consider within the narratives that represent today's health care and educational milieu who our trainees are, what our optimal learning environments should look like, and what our curricula – explicit as well as tacit – should include.

A growing number of articles in the literature note significant generational differences between current medical students and residents and their predecessors. Johnston has described the current generation of trainees and young physicians, *Generation X,* as having a number of characteristics which are important to consider as we focus our educational strategies toward them. She points out that these physicians (22: 188):

> . . . were raised during a period of unprecedented rapid social change . . ., experienced a significant shift in traditional family structure, entered increasingly diverse social networks . . . adapted to the rapid access to endless information available in their homes through desktop technology . . ., [and] saw their parents subjected to corporate downsizing and the dissolution of institutional loyalty.

In addition, a number of authors report that this generation is more focused on protecting their personal lives and balancing personal needs with their professional obligations (22, 26, 27). "Accordingly", Johnston (22: 188) elaborates, "the concept of altruism which can conflict with desire for a controllable lifestyle, or more time for a personal life, is a concept being negotiated by the new generation." To emphasize this point, perhaps even to suggest a degree of alarm about it, Hafferty (27) tells the story of his experiences teaching first-year medical students at his institution, reporting that they rejected the belief that they were under any obligation whatsoever in medicine. He went on to describe their strong desire for *balance* that would allow them to appropriately attend to their personal and family lives. These students also objected to the expectation that they would be held to the higher standards of the profession, stating that they had not *signed on* to any such expectations before entering medical school. They acknowledged the existence of professional standards, but did not feel compelled to commit to them. Contemporary students, in Hafferty's observations, have begun to construct a new storyline – one in which the work of medicine is balanced with the needs of its practitioners, and in which obligations are set internally and individually, rather than by the external forces of the profession itself or the community.

If these characterizations hold true of our newest generation of students and physicians, consciousness of such beliefs and tendencies ought to inform our educational efforts. A didactic model of professionalism education – an attempt to simply educate about *how it is* – is less likely to be successful than a narrative that engages students and residents with stories of profession, meaningful self-reflection, and debate around what we might agree to be contemporary professionalism portraits. As Stanley Joel Reiser (28: 4) has pointed out, ". . . all teaching involves the simultaneous transmission of two lessons [narratives]: one is a lesson about theory or technique – why nature or artifact is what it is, or how to do something; the second is a lesson about ethics – the teacher's response to the student's effort to learn and grow" (insertion added). Recognizing these two landscapes of teaching – technical and ethical (not dissimilar to Bruner's story landscapes described in Chapter 4) – requires educators to be as concerned with what and why ideas are transmitted as with how content is taught. In addition, educators will need to expend greater energy focusing on the *culture* of medical education as much as its curricular content since, as Reiser comments (28: 4), ". . . diminishing the significance of concern and respect in human relationships may be by far the most powerful lesson that teachers leave behind."

Trainee engagement in the content and character of their own education will continue to be critical as the next generation's narratives of *professionalism* are constructed. Mary Anne Johnston (29: 96) comments that "Students themselves are grappling with the definition of professionalism in an age when static conceptions of 'core values' may not lead to the development of such values or attributes in medical students." In describing examples of students who actively sought to influence their own professionalism curricula in response to their own concerns about current health care issues, she proposes that medical students can become critically important resources for their own professional development.

In considering what should be taught, and in what kinds of learning environments, Jack Coulehan describes a narrative approach (30: 24):

For professionalism to mold behavior, it has to be articulated as a meta-narrative, a summation of, and reflection upon, many thousands of stories of actual physicians in different times and cultures, including contemporary narratives observed directly through role model physicians and other health professionals and indirectly through stories and film. In other words, to learn professionalism is to enter into a certain level of narrative and make it one's own. I call this *narrative professionalism*. It has been diluted or missing in medical education for some time.

Elsewhere, Coulehan and colleagues (31: 30) propose that a professionalism curriculum would need to offer cognitive and experiential learning opportunities in the following four essential elements: ". . . (1) personal reflection and reflective practice; (2) narrative competence; (3) strong role model engagement and interaction; and (4) community service."

In support of Coulehan's proposed curriculum, we would expand upon some of the elements he includes and suggest the following for undergraduate and graduate medical education in our institutions. These recommendations begin to construct a storyline within medical education that is more responsive to the moral and spiritual presence of the practitioner – to moral and spiritual *agency* as critically important in caregiving.

First, throughout our curricula, there should be regular and structured opportunities, with guidance by appropriate faculty, for trainees to reflect on their own development. To that end, a number of medical schools and residency programs have begun to incorporate narrative activities such as reflective writing, small group discussions, storytelling, and engagement with imaginative literature. For example, at Northeastern Ohio Universities College of Medicine, as part of a complete transformation of our curriculum, faculty have created within a longitudinal *Doctoring* course regular small group sessions, beginning in the first year, in which students meet with faculty preceptors, basic science and clinical faculty together, to discuss their reactions to selected writings, stories, articles, film, and poetry. The topics are chosen to have relevance to the student's particular stage of development, and include, among others, cheating and honor codes, gender issues, substance abuse and impairment, and emotion in medicine. For each session the students are expected to submit in advance of the meeting a reflective essay that discusses what the assigned readings mean to them with regard to their own development as physicians.

One of our first-year students, in the early months of his medical school career, wrote the following poem in response to assigned readings related to his cadaver experience. The discussion sessions were held during the anatomy course.

A Letter to My Cadaver With Some Questions I Still Have

Dear
Mr {...}:

Did you
    Hesitate?
(Because I would have
– Ten or
Thirty times.)

Did you like science
When you were
Young?

    Who was your favorite teacher?

Cream with your coffee?
What are your
Top five
Favorite songs?
Sunset or sunrise? Ever
Find it hard
Just to
Sleep?

Did you ever
Find your true
Love?

When did you know?

Tell me about
You.
Please.
(There is so much I don't know.)

Thank you.

Ramon Cancino

This student is as conscious about the work he is doing with his cadaver as he is about what that work means. Related to the narrative landscapes discussed in Chapter 4, he is operating in the action landscape in the anatomy lab, and in the consciousness landscape that resides in his cadaver as person.

Secondly, *safe space* must be created throughout our curricula where trainees can step back from their daily work and explore the implications of their experiences for their own development as physicians. This is particularly true during clinical training. Students typically experience great moral turbulence during their education, related to the contradictions mentioned earlier between what they have been taught about professionalism and what they see enacted in real-world medicine narratives. They come to learn, through what has been described as the *hidden curriculum,* how it really is. They are compelled to get in step, to assimilate into the real world of medicine. They often sublimate their own moral urges not to assimilate, fearing recrimination if they go against the grain – recrimination that could hamper their academic advancement. And they may succumb to what we described earlier as a sense of powerlessness informed by their belief that even if they were to speak out to express their different, perhaps more idealistic views and to report inappropriate events they witness or are forced to partake in, nothing will come of their reporting. We need to provide them with some safety which might allow them to stand on moral ground, and some reason to trust that we will respond appropriately to their concerns.

Thirdly, open and guided conversations with our residents, nurses, and attending physicians are necessary to discuss how their words and actions give shape to their trainees' professional identities and behaviors. We need to support positive role models in their stress-filled environments in ways that encourage them to spend more time in the politically difficult moral high ground. And we need to nurture and reward the best role models.

Fourthly, academic institutions must reconstruct the narratives within their own *cultures,* and collectively share stories which demonstrate that they are indeed moral communities as well as healing communities. Colleagues at the Indiana University School of Medicine have made impressive strides in *changing the conversations* at their own institution. Through their relationship-centered care initiative, they have created ways to engage all participants in the medical education enterprise to explore in more conscious ways what is happening to them. Through appreciative inquiry strategies, they are finding ways to move in the direction of *being at their best* in terms of how they work with patients, and how they work with each other (see Further Activities section).

Fifthly, curricula should be structured in ways that allow students to know that competence includes both logico-scientific and narrative competence. It is here that we would make a case for a broader definition of competence, one that honors the complementary role of both forms. The competency-based curriculum movement currently under way in medical education offers hope here. As educators place communication, professionalism, self-awareness, and reflective practice on a par with medical knowledge and clinical skill, it is conceivable that statements such as "He's a good doctor but he can't talk to his patients" will be recognized as incongruous and contradictory.

Sixthly, medical educators need to remain sensitive to the many connotations of the *P word.* This narrative concept was discussed earlier in the chapter. Perhaps what is needed is for teachers and learners together to co-construct a new narrative definition of professionalism that could mitigate its negative connotations.

Finally, as we consider the environments in which young health care professionals develop their professional identities, we ought to demonstrate how serious we are about the precepts we teach by how they are enacted within our curricula. John Saultz (32) has suggested that if teaching institutions are serious about professionalism teaching, they should consider making changes in their learning environments which would support the following initiatives:

- address cost and access to care as first-order intellectual problems
- humanize science and restore scientific integrity beyond the requirements of compliance programs
- celebrate those who best embody moral leadership in our profession
- acknowledge and take responsibility for the relationship and the practice choices of our graduates and the availability of affordable health care to our people.

During a presentation at our institution, Jack Coulehan shared one of his poems, written for the Stony Brook Medical School Class of 1994, entitled *Turning the Page*. He expressed a desire, with which we concur, for a new narrative of professionalism that would invite young professionals to enter a world of service in medicine in which they can fulfill their dreams of truly caring for others as healers (33: 26):

Turning the Page

This is not the end. It's where
the story takes a twist
like when your palms turned moist
on being sent to see the ill
not just with eyes, but with
your heart as well. It's where the tale
takes an unexpected turn, a turn
you might *expect* but not
exactly now – slogging through
the wilderness of words
you've searched for years,
you find the track your quarry left –
it's near! It's where
the hero comes, of course
galloping high across the page
and where you find the hero's name
is yours. This is not the end.
It's where the champion charges in
to kill the dragon, save the day.
She doesn't fail.
This is the page where you come in
to tell the tale.

Jack Coulehan

NARRATIVE IN THE PRACTITIONER–COMMUNITY DIMENSION
The Narrative of Medicine as Community

A number of years ago, a visiting professor at our institution told a story that continues to resonate in our work today. He described an experience he had while presenting a community program attended by lay people on the topic of how to achieve balance in the rapid-paced, hectic lives that are so common in our society. He had wandered into a conversation about the concept of *community*, and was engaging his audience in an effort to describe what *community* meant to them. He noticed an Amish man in a wide-brimmed hat who had been silent during the entire seminar while most others had participated in the conversation. Deciding to take a risk, he approached the man, asking him if he would mind describing his sense of community to the group. The man piously rose to his feet, removed his hat and gently placed it on his chair, turned to the group and spoke. Our recollection of what the Amish man was reported to have said follows:

> In the early morning hours, my son and I go out to plow our fields. From the vantage point of our farm as we look across the broad horizon, we can see seventeen other farms where other farmers are out with their sons, plowing their fields. And I know that if today I step into a hole and twist my ankle or break my leg, tomorrow my field will still get plowed.

The man then turned, placed his hat back on his head, and sat down. Our visitor described the silence which followed the man's remarks as the rest of the audience considered what he had said.

This man's conceptualization of community is one we earnestly long for, both in our work world and in the broader world in which we live. It is an essence of community that describes the difference between living in the world *with* each other and living in the world *for* each other. People who live with this man's sense of community, believe in it and act on it, are likely to manifest a considerable degree of *other-directedness*, a disposition toward *other* that is central to altruism and an ethic of service. If altruism and generosity can be considered to be critical characteristics of professionalism, if not its central characteristics, then this formulation of community should loom large in the health care professions both in how caregivers relate to each other, and in how they relate to their communities.

Communities are inherently narrative structures. As Lewis and Sandra Hinchman have described (2: 238), "It is narratives, along with the values they describe, that form the basis of communities large and small, and thereby define who we are. . . . We extend or withhold allegiance to communities depending on our rational judgments concerning the narratives on which they are based." The profession of medicine as a community comprises a rich set of narratives describing its origins, its goals and obligations, its values, and its development. Even on a smaller scale, within individual practices or health care settings, the narratives of medical work form *communities of presence*, or *communities of caring* as Charon has described them (25). "If pastoral care connects suffering individuals with communities of faith, and trauma care connects individual trauma survivors with communities of survivors and witnesses", Charon points out (25: 198), ". . . then narrative medicine can connect patients and their caregivers with their natural communities of care."

Contemporary medicine has come under criticism, as we have been describing, for the extent to which it has often failed to live up to its obligations as a community. In these ways, medicine's functioning as a community has been disrupted. Walter Fisher (34: 322) has written about:

> . . . how communities . . . such as medicine and law, become corrupt
> when their practitioners pursue values external to them. When doctors
> and lawyers pursue money, power, and prestige to the detriment of
> health and justice, their professions suffer and so do their characters,
> at least within those professions by those who still adhere to the ideals
> that constitute the practice.

Fisher's observations describe the consequences of such *corruption*, both to the profession and to the individual practitioner. This is descriptive of a tension that resides in the physician–profession domain, since as MacIntyre states (35: 259), ". . . the self has to find its moral identity in and through its membership in communities", but is not expected to be extinguished by virtue of its membership. The particularity of a given member's identity can never be extinguished. So within a community such as medicine, individual members are expected to uphold the values and fulfill the obligations of that community individually, and they are expected to work toward ensuring that the community is loyal to these values and obligations as well.

The profession's narrative identity is not a static one. Communities like medicine reinvent or re-story themselves continuously, and do so through the use of what Fisher (34: 320) calls *reaffirmative rhetoric*, whose ". . . characteristic forms are arguments reasserting the validity of the community's creed or modes of ceremonial, communal transactions." This process of reaffirmation, through telling and re-telling, is protective. In Richard Kearney's view (36: 249), communities:

> . . . which admit that they constitute themselves through an ongoing
> process of narrative are unlikely to degenerate into self-righteousness,
> . . . that is the capacity of narrative imagination constantly to transcend
> the status quo of any given society toward possible alternatives that
> sustains a sense of ethical attentiveness to others.

Yet, as mentioned previously, physicians individually and the medical profession collectively have been criticized for actions and positions which contradict their commitments to ethically attend to others. A number of forces divide physicians, disrupt the *community-ness* of medicine, and challenge the precepts of professionalism. Perhaps foremost among these forces is the shift from medicine's identity as a calling to one more consistent with that of a business – from a professional culture of service provision to a commercial one (11). Pellegrino laments these developments (37: 383):

> Unfortunately, today many professional associations are preoccupied with financial survival, corporate growth, investment strategies, benefits for members, fees for testimonials, etc. There is little energy left for promulgation of the ethical purposes of the profession as a professor. In these respects professional medical associations seem to justify the opinions of the Federal Trade Commission, which classifies medicine primarily as a business and not as an ethical entity.

Other forces have served to diminish medicine's functioning as a community, and the literature is replete with their descriptions. P Preston Reynolds (38) cites medicine's increasing specialization, the manner in which heath care economics have led to increased service demands on residents, and the systems in place to reward faculty as some of the forces that have disrupted the medical education community, and thus threatened professionalism. In addition to the movement toward a business model of medicine, John Saultz (32) identifies the growing number of people who cannot access health care as medicine's most pressing moral crisis, and also describes the deterioration of trust in the academic community that has resulted from increasingly public scandals within our research institutions, citing these narratives as disruptive to the concept of professionalism. A more comprehensive list of issues that divide physicians, diminish medicine as a community, and challenge the tenets of professionalism comes from Hafferty and Light (5), and can be summarized as follows:

- specialization, and specialty battles over qualifications to do procedures
- turf battles among specialists and primary care physicians
- capitation payment arrangements, reducing specialty referrals
- Medicare's resource-based relative value scale (RBRVS) payment methodologies
- work hour limits for trainees
- health care reform debates
- physician ownership of health care-related facilities and "conflict of interest" issues
- lack of self-policing within medicine
- corporate and governmental influences on health care
- proliferation of other health care providers.

Although this list is not exhaustive, it is clear that many contemporary issues facing medicine serve to divide its members, and diminish the extent to which medicine functions as a community.

John Gardner (39: 5), former secretary of Health, Education and Welfare, wrote a powerful document, *Building Community*, in which he describes communities as ". . . the ground-level generators and preservers of values and ethical systems. No society can remain vital or even survive without a reasonable base of shared values." His description (39: 7) of the place of communities in contemporary society bears relevance to the discussion of medicine as a community:

> Progressively the traditional community has been stripped of its autonomy and deprived of many of its functions. Today we see the weakening and collapse of communities, of obligations and commitment, and of coherent belief systems. We see a loss of a sense of identity and belonging, of opportunities for allegiance, for being needed and responding to need – and a corresponding rise in feelings of alienation, impotence, and anomie.

In addition, Gardner observes that traditional communities have shifted from being quite homogeneous to ever increasing heterogeneity, from unchanging to welcoming change, from being characterized by conformity to cultures of pluralism and adaptation, from isolated stances to greater connectedness with the world around them, from exclusivity of membership to inclusivity, and from organizations with great continuity and long histories to processes of continual re-storying. Many of these cultural shifts have had implications for medicine, and have influenced medicine's responses to many of the above-mentioned challenges to its integrity as a profession.

Gardner outlines ten attributes of communities, and admits that he did so with the specific intention of allowing assessment of any given institution or social system regarding whether it truly functions as a community. The attributes are summarized below (39: 15–26):

Ten Attributes of Community

1 Wholeness incorporating diversity
2 Reasonable base of shared values
3 Caring, trust, and teamwork
4 Effective internal communication
5 Participation
6 Affirmation
7 Links beyond the community
8 Development of young people
9 A forward view
10 Institutional arrangements for community maintenance

We were unable to resist the temptation to consider these ten attributes in the context of medicine as a community. Is medicine's story a narrative of community?

With regard to *diversity*, it is conceivable that one aspect of medicine's diversity, manifested by a storyline of increasing specialization and sub-specialization, has been to its detriment. This may be in part because, as a profession, medicine has not followed Gardner's suggestion (39: 16) that it should develop ". . . institutional arrangements for diminishing polarization, for teaching diverse groups to know one another, for coalition-building, dispute resolution, negotiation and mediation." Restoring this sense of community in medicine will require all of its constituencies to reaffirm their commitments to service and align around those commitments.

In another dimension of diversity, numerous efforts to increase the racial and ethnic diversity of the profession have met with suboptimal success. Long-term investments have been made in pipeline programs and other initiatives aimed at enhancing the applicant pool to support these diversity initiatives. There is hope that these efforts will enjoy more long-term success. In any dimension, diversity is a laudable goal for medicine, as Gardner points out, not just as a way of broadening tolerance within a community, but also as a way to ensure greater adaptability and renewal in an ever changing world.

There is little doubt that medicine's narrative is founded upon a *reasonable base of shared values*, which Gardner believes to be the most important of the ten attributes. What has led to criticisms of the profession is the extent to which its members live (or don't live) these values in the work, and the extent to which the profession's initiatives are aligned with these values. A community that enjoys shared values is also responsible for transmitting them to its current and future members. A healthy community, Gardner posits (39: 17), ". . . will impart a coherent value system. If it is chaotic or degenerate, lessons will be taught anyway – but not lessons that heal or strengthen." The concerns raised in this chapter and in Chapter 4 regarding our medical education challenges support this claim and suggest an *unhealthy* community. In many respects, the push toward narrative forms of medical practice and narrative education and competence is in part a response to failure of the community of medicine to sustain its values in practice and in teaching. If medicine is to regain its ability to function as a community, it will have to meet this challenge, as has been so eloquently stated by Gardner (39: 17):

> . . . most future communities will have to build and continuously repair the framework of shared values. Their norms will have to be explicitly taught. Values that are never expressed are apt to be taken for granted and not adequately conveyed to young people and newcomers. Individuals have a role in the continuous rebuilding of the value framework, and the best thing that they can do is not to preach values but to exemplify them. Teach the truth by living it.

Caring, trust, and teamwork have been inconsistently enacted within the narrative of medicine. The divides described earlier have diminished medicine's sense of *team*, and as we have discussed earlier, students and residents who enter the world of clinical medicine, hopeful for a life of service to the suffering, do not always encounter caring environments, either directed toward patients or toward themselves. Yet, as Gardner has pointed out (39: 18):

> . . . members of a good community deal with one another humanely, respect individual differences and value the integrity of each person. A good community fosters an atmosphere of cooperation and connectedness. There is recognition and thanks for hard work, and an awareness by the members that they need one another. There is a sense of belonging and identity, a spirit of mutual responsibility.

With regard to *communication* and *participation*, it could be said that too many physicians fail to fulfill the obligation to participate in, or to *serve*, their profession. Nor are such expectations explicit in the training of our newest physicians. However, as Gardner suggests (39: 11), "Passive allegiance isn't enough today. The forces of disintegration have gained steadily and will prevail unless individuals see themselves as having a positive duty to nurture their community and continuously reweave the social fabric." The process of *reaffirmation* is clearly enacted throughout the rituals, celebrations, and oath-taking practices of medical education and the profession of medicine. And as we have described previously, new physicians affirm their commitments while provoking new ways of thinking about the profession and its obligations. This continual reassessment and re-emplotment is a healthy process for the community of medicine. "The process of renewal", Gardner states (39: 11), ". . . encompasses both continuity and change, reinterpreting tradition to meet new conditions, building a better future on an acknowledged heritage and the wisdom of experience. That calls for loving, nurturing critics."

Of greater concern, we might argue, is whether the profession can sustain a sense of obligation and duty on the part of its members, especially in view of what have been described as emerging attitudes of contemporary medical students in this regard (27). However, to the extent that medicine is a profession built upon the application of specialized knowledge and skills in service to others, these tenets of professionalism are inarguable.

In making the argument for a community *to build connections outside of itself*, Gardner (39) cautions that communities need to resist becoming insular, for that condition decreases connections with others. Medicine's most formidable challenge may be to continue to re-emplot its relationships with the people and communities that it is meant to serve, and in so doing, to recommit to a narrative of trust. As a community, medicine will need to focus, first and foremost, on shifting away from its storyline of self-serving business motivations back to one that demonstrates more altruistic motivations in order to succeed at this rebuilding. In addition, Gardner (39) warns that a community must protect its members from external forces that erode its integrity. Clearly, medicine's troubled relationships with industry need to be addressed as a priority for the profession. On this issue, leadership in academic medicine has begun to emerge in policy proposals (40) and among academic health centers that are beginning to address these concerns, and their efforts must build momentum across the profession to construct new narratives wherever care is delivered or taught.

With regard to Gardner's final three attributes – the *development of young people*, a *forward view*, and *institutional arrangements for community maintenance* – we believe that there may be cause for optimism. Educational institutions, both at the undergraduate level and in graduate medical education, have begun to focus efforts on ways to reinvigorate professionalism in its future members. Charon's idea of a *narrative federation*, as described in Chapter 4, is likely to be a force for better education in the humanistic practices of medicine.

Today, against the ten attributes outlined by Gardner, medicine does not score high marks as a community. However, a forward-looking narrative for the profession, if re-emplotted with the essential commitments of medicine as the profession's highest priorities, offers hope of a reaffirmation of the profession, and a rebuilding of medicine's narrative as one of community.

Narrative in a Broader Social Context

While we have been discussing the concept of community, we have done so in the context of *profession* as community. We have discussed the extent to which the narrative of medicine as profession is a narrative of community. We now turn to a different context of community. We shall address the narrative dimensions of the broader community and society, and the practitioner's role within that context as it relates to narrative work.

Narrative medical practice is a community engagement. While the traditional focus of health care has been on the care of individual patients, Coulehan and Williams (41: 53) point out that ". . . meeting this responsibility often requires attention to the social environment from which the patient comes and to which he or she returns. In this sense *some* attention to social context has always been derivatively necessary." As we come to understand our patients' narratives, we come to operate inside their particular communities, and in the narratives of those communities, in our efforts to heal. In addition, as health care practitioners, we become part of the communities in which our patients participate, and we in fact create communities – *communities of presence*, as described by Charon (25). Even in death we make connections with our patients and their communities. Patrick Irvine, a physician in St Paul, Minnesota, wrote about his experiences attending his patients' funerals (42: 1705):

> In a special way, it gives me perhaps my best understanding of how that person fit into his or her community, and how medical care fit into that life – on the patient's own ground rather than my medical ground

– away from the demeaning patient gowns, the sterile professional uniforms, and the white lights of the intensive-care unit. The funeral brings that person back home to the community to rest; we are part of that community too.

In an even broader context, there is the obligation for practitioners to concern themselves with the health of communities as well as with that of individual patients. The American Medical Association's (43) principles of medical ethics include the responsibility to actively contribute to improving community and public health, as well as an expectation of supporting access to health care for everyone. Russell Gruen and colleagues at the Harvard School of Public Health present compelling reasons for physicians to become more actively engaged in public health issues (44: 94):

> First, community socioeconomic characteristics affect many health problems and access to health care; second, physicians' expertise is essential for properly addressing major quality, access, public health, and policy concerns; and third, clear and visible leadership in the interests of the public's health is regarded by many as the best way for the medical profession to regain and retain the public trust that has diminished in recent decades . . .

Table 5.1 Social Contract between Medicine and Society (45: 171)

Society's Expectations of Medicine	Medicine's Expectations of Society
Services of the healer	Trust
Assured competence	Autonomy
Altruistic service	Self-regulation
Morality and integrity	Health care system
	– value-driven
Accountability	– adequately funded
Transparency	Participation in public policy
Source of objective advice	Shared responsibility for health (patients and society)
Promotion of the public good	Monopoly
	Status and rewards
	– non-financial: respect and status
	– financial

Many medical schools have community health components in their curricula to expose students to the ways in which public health affects individual health, and how these issues can be addressed. These educational narratives are in support of what has been described as medicine's contract with society.

Sylvia Creuss has described the essential elements of that contract, which are summarized in Table 5.1.

It is useful to consider the implications for narrative work in fulfilling the obligations attendant on this social contact. Each of society's expectations, as outlined in Creuss's tabulation, is supported by narrative practice. As Rita Charon (25) has pointed out, the narrative projects that were begun at Columbia can have a real impact on the quality improvement initiatives of the health system through interaction with administrative and planning personnel. She believes that (25: 228):

> . . . narrative medicine training . . . can make contributions to patient-centered and timely health care by providing cost-effective, integrated, and boundary-crossing methods of inspecting and valuing health care professionals' work within climates of trust and collaboration. By contributing to the well-being of individual health professionals, the cohesiveness of teams, the sustained and disciplined recognition of patients' and family's perspectives, and the circulation of knowledge and information outside of traditional silos of health care systems, narrative training can provide hospital staff with new clinical skills, personal reward, heightened stake in the mission, and the fortifying trust that their work matters. At the same time, narrative work may help to level the stratified hierarchy of the health care setting. Our growth in narrative capacities may enable us recognize damaging power relationships within our hospital and help us choose to work toward fair and equitable professional collaboration in the care of the sick.

She goes on to point out in more global terms that *knowledge of the other*, obtained through narrative practices, can contribute to a broader understanding of suffering and health and contribute to healthier communities. "Because of the ethical duties the listener incurs by virtue of having heard personal reports of trauma or pain", Charon (25: 232) concludes, "the communities that result from such ways of knowing are moral communities as well as clinical communities."

FURTHER ACTIVITIES

1 Stories resulting from an appreciative inquiry process may be found at http://meded.iusm.iu.edu. At this site select "Reflecting Caring Attitudes Through Action – 2006 RCCI Publication."

REFERENCES

1 George D, Gonsenhauser I, Whitehouse P. Medical professionalism: the nature of story and the story of nature. In: Wear D, Aultman JM, editors. *Professionalism in Medicine: critical perspectives.* New York: Springer; 2006. pp. 63–86.

2 Hinchman LP, Hinchman SK, editors. *Memory, Identity, Community: the idea of narrative in the human sciences.* New York: State University of New York Press; 2001.

3 Creuss RL, Cruess SR, Johnston SE. Renewing professionalism: an opportunity for medicine. *Acad Med.* 1999; **74:** 878–84.

4 Cruess RL, Cruess SR. Teaching medicine as a profession in the service of healing. *Acad Med.* 1997; **72:** 941–52.

5 Hafferty FW, Light DW. Professional dynamics and the changing nature of medical work. *J Health Soc Behav.* 1995; **35:** 132–53.

6 Brandeis L. *Business: a profession.* Boston, MA: Small, Olaguard; 1914.

7 Friedson E. *Professional Dominance: the social structure of medical care.* Chicago: Aldine; 1970.

8 Haug MR. Deprofessionalization: an alternate hypothesis for the future. *Sociol Rev Monograph.* 1973; **20:** 195–211.

9 McKinlay JB, Arches J. Toward the proletarianization of physicians. *Int J Health Serv.* 1985; **15:** 161–95.

10 Starr P. *The Social Transformation of American Medicine; the rise of a sovereign profession and the making of a vast industry.* New York: Basic Books; 1982.

11 McArthur JH, Moore FD. The two cultures and the health care revolution: commerce and professionalism in medical care. *JAMA.* 1997; **277:** 985–9.

12 Committee on Quality of Health Care in America, Institute of Medicine. *Crossing the Quality Chasm: a new health system for the 21st century.* Washington. DC: National Academies Press; 2001.

13 Smedley BD, Stith AY, Nelson AR, editors. *Unequal Treatment: confronting racial and ethnic disparities in health care.* Washington, DC: National Academies Press; 2003.

14 Gibbs N, Bower A. Q: What scares doctors? A: Being the patient. *Time.* 2006; **1 May:** 43–52.

15 Castellani B, Hafferty FW. The complexities of medical professionalism: a preliminary investigation. In: Wear D, Aultman JM, editors. *Professionalism in Medicine: critical perspectives.* New York: Springer; 2006. pp. 3–23.

16 Inui TS. *A Flag in the Wind: educating for professionalism in medicine.* Washington, DC: American Association of Medical Colleges; 2003.

17 Association of American Medical Colleges Graduation Questionnaire; www.aamc. org/data/gq/allschoolsreports/2006.pdf

18 Wear D, Aultman JM, Varley JD *et al.* Making fun of patients: medical students' perceptions and use of derogatory and cynical humor in clinical settings. *Acad Med.* 2006; **81:** 454–62.

19 Medical Professionalism Project. Medical professionalism in the new millennium: a physician's charter. *Lancet.* 2002; **359:** 520–22.

20 American Board of Internal Medicine (ABIM) Foundation, American College of Physicians – American Society of Internal Medicine (ACP-ASIM) Foundation and European Federation of Internal Medicine. Medical professionalism in the new millennium: a physician charter. *Ann Intern Med.* 2002; **136:** 243–6.

21 Coulehan J. You say self-interest, I say altruism. In: Wear D, Aultman JM, editors. *Professionalism in Medicine: critical perspectives.* New York: Springer; 2006. pp. 103–27.

22 Johnston S. See one, do one, teach one: developing professionalism across the generations. *Clin Orthop Relat Res.* 2006; **449:** 186–92.

23 Connelly JE. The other side of professionalism: doctor-to-doctor. *Camb Q Healthcare Ethics*. 2003; **12:** 178–83.

24 Hafferty FW. Definitions of professionalism: a search for meaning and identity. *Clin Orthop Relat Res*. 2006; **449:** 193–204.

25 Charon R. *Narrative Medicine: honoring the stories of illness*. Oxford: Oxford University Press; 2006.

26 Smith LG. Medical professionalism and the generation gap. *Am J Med*. 2005; **118:** 439–42.

27 Hafferty FW. What medical students know about professionalism. *Mt Sinai J Med*. 2002; **69:** 385–97.

28 Reiser SJ. The moral order of the medical school. In: Wear D, Bickel J, editors. *Educating for Professionalism: creating a culture of humanism in medical education*. Iowa City, IA: University of Iowa Press; 2000. pp. 3–10.

29 Johnston MAC. Reflections on experiences with socially active students. In: Wear D, Bickel J, editors. *Educating For Professionalism: creating a culture of humanism in medical education*. Iowa City, IA: University of Iowa Press; 2000. pp. 95–104.

30 Coulehan J. I witness, I serve: medicine as community. In: *Proceedings of the Fourth Humanism and the Healing Arts Conference. Institute for Professionalism Inquiry*. Akron, OH: Summa Health System; 2006.

31 Coulehan J, Williams PC, Van McCrary S *et al*. The best lack all conviction: biomedical ethics, professionalism, and social responsibility. *Camb Q Healthcare Ethics*. 2003; **12:** 21–38.

32 Saultz JW. Are we serious about teaching professionalism in medicine? *Acad Med*. 2007; **82:** 574–7.

33 Coulehan J. Turning the page. In: *The Heavenly Ladder*. Canberra: Ginninderra Press; 2001. p. 26.

34 Fisher WR. Narration, reason, and community. In: Hinchman LP, Hinchman SK, editors. *Memory, Identity, and Community: the idea of narrative in the human sciences*. Albany, NY: State University of New York Press; 2001. pp. 307–27.

35 MacIntyre A. The virtues, the unity of a human life, and the concept of a tradition. In: Hinchman LP, Hinchman SK, editors. *Memory, Identity, and Community: the idea of narrative in the human sciences*. Albany, NY: State University of New York Press; 2001. pp. 241–63.

36 Kearney R. *Poetics of Imagining: modern to post-modern*. New York: Fordham University Press; 1998.

37 Pellegrino ED. Professionalism, profession and the virtues of a good physician. *Mt Sinai J Med*. 2002; **69:** 378–84.

38 Reynolds PP. Reaffirming professionalism through the education community. *Ann Intern Med*. 1994; **120:** 609–14.

39 Gardner JW. *Building Community*. Washington, DC: Independent Sector; 1991.

40 Brennan TA, Rothman DJ, Blank L *et al*. Health industry practices that create conflicts of interest: a policy proposal for academic medical centers. *JAMA*. 2006; **295:** 429–33.

41 Coulehan J, Williams PC. Professional ethics and social activism. Where have we been? Where are we going? In: Wear D, Bickel J, editors. *Educating for Professionalism: creating a culture of humanism in medical education*. Iowa City IA: University of Iowa Press; 2000. pp. 49–69.

42 Irvine P. The attending at the funeral. *NEJM*. 1985; **312**: 1704–5.

43 American Medical Association. *Principles of Medical Ethics*, www.ama-assn.org/ama/ pub/category/2512.html

44 Gruen RL, Pearson SD, Brennan TA. Physician-citizens – public roles and professional obligations. *JAMA*. 2004; **291**: 94–8.

45 Cruess SR. Professionalism and medicine's social contract with society. *Clin Orthop Relat Res*. 2006; **449**: 170–76.

INTERLUDE

We have provided this pause between Part 2 and the remaining sections of the book to provide an example of medical readers' theater – an activity that uses stories, specifically plays, in narrative skill training. We have chosen to adapt Leo Tolstoy's widely read classic novella, *The Death of Ivan Ilyich*, as a play. We describe the use of medical readers' theater in Chapter 6.

The Death of Ivan Ilyich*

by
Leo Tolstoy

CAST

****

Narrator
Ivan Ilyich Golovin
Praskovya Feodorovna Golovin (Ivan's wife)
Elizaveta (Liza) (Ivan's daughter)
Vassili (Ivan's son – no spoken part)
Gerasim (houseservant)
Lacofsky (Praskovya's brother)
Piotr Ivanovich (colleague)
Feodor Vassilievich (colleague)
Leschititsky (eminent doctor)
Nikolayev (ordinary doctor)

Scene 1

Narrator: The time and setting for our story is nineteenth-century Russia. We begin our story by hearing about Ivan Ilyich Golovin's life and career in the years preceding his death.

For many years since his graduation from law school Ivan Ilyich had enjoyed a highly successful professional life as a magistrate of the courts, with continual promotions and assignments in various locations. At the time of his death he was serving in Petersburg.

Early in his career Ivan had married Praskovya Feodorovna Mikhel, who came from good aristocratic stock and was sweet, intelligent, pretty, and eminently respectable. The beginning of their married life was blissful until Praskovya first became pregnant, and with the birth of additional children she grew increasingly jealous, demanding of his attention, and disagreeable and

---

* Adapted from *The Death Of Ivan Ilyich And Master Of Man* by Leo Tolstoy, translated by Ann Pasternak Slater, copyright © 2003 by Ann Pasternak Slater. Used by permission of Modern Library, a division of Random House, Inc.

generally disruptive of their pleasant lifestyle. The deaths of two of their children severely compounded the situation. The more irritating and demanding his wife became, the more Ivan transferred the center of gravity of his life to his work, and the more ambitious he became. Soon his life focused on his work, the consciousness of his own power and the importance of his success in the eyes of high and low. Unfortunately, still another child died, leaving only his daughter, Elizaveta, now sixteen, and his young schoolboy son, Vassili. So it was that Ivan lived for several more years.

We now move forward to the time following Ivan's death. At the news of his death, Ivan's colleagues, who knew he had been ill for several weeks with an incurable disease, began thinking of their own probable career advancements now that a vacancy had opened. The closest of his friends were Vassilievich and Ivanovich.

Feodor Vassilievich: Now I'll probably get Shtabel's place or Vinnikov's. It's been promised to me for a long time. What exactly was wrong with Ivan Ilyich?

Piotr Ivanovich: Each of his doctors thought something different. The last time I saw him, I thought he'd get better. Yes, now that he is gone, I'll have to put in for my brother-in-law's transfer from Kaluga. My wife will be very pleased, and no one can say I never did anything for her relatives. But since I have been friends with Ivan since law school, I feel an obligation to him. I will attend his funeral.

Narrator: Just before the funeral was to begin, Praskovya took Ivanovich aside.

Praskovya: I know that you were a true friend to Ivan Ilyich. I must have a word with you. Ivan Ilyich suffered dreadfully in his last days. Oh, it was terrible! For three days on end he screamed without stopping. It was unbearable. I can't understand how I survived it. My God, how I suffered.

Narrator: Ivanovich thought to himself.

Ivanovich: Three days of appalling suffering and death. Why, that could happen to me too, at any time. But thinking such thoughts is not good for me. I must think of other things.

Narrator: Weeping, Praskovya continued to speak to Ivanovich of her primary concern, which was how she could wring more money out of the Treasury on her husband's death. Ivanovich believed that nothing more could be done.

When Ivanovich entered the funeral room he met Ivan's beautiful young daughter, Elizaveta. She was dressed in black and wore a gloomy, almost angry expression. Behind her stood her fiancé, also a magistrate – a wealthy young man with a similarly offended expression. Ivanovich then caught sight of Ivan's small schoolboy son. He saw that Vassili's eyes were tearstained.

Narrator: When Ivan and his family had first arrived in Petersburg, they had secured an excellent apartment, exactly what he and his wife had dreamed of. He personally oversaw the decorations, and at times did some of the decorating himself. On just such an occasion, he fell off a ladder and hit his side against the handle of a window. It hurt for a little while but the pain then passed. The new apartment had a distinctly aristocratic flavour, and they had all settled into a harmonious life and courted members of the proper social class at their new home.

Scene 2

Narrator: When Ivan Ilyich's illness first began, he complained of a strange taste in his mouth and something that felt not quite right on the left side of his stomach. Then the discomfort began to increase – not quite pain, but an awareness of a permanent heaviness in his side. He fell into a poor state of mind which grew stronger and began to spoil the light and much more pleasant way of life just established in the Golovin household. Now it was he who most often started the quarrelling, and generally this was at the moment he started eating. He began to blame Praskovya for everything.

Praskovya: Ivan Ilyich, it is fortunate that I was blessed with such a sweet nature to put up with your difficult character and horrible temper all these years. As for your illness, I believe you must have a constitutional disorder prompted by food.

Narrator: Praskovya decided that her husband's appalling character made her life a misery, and the more she pitied herself, the more she loathed her husband. She started wishing that he would die, but realized that if he did die there would be no salary and that made her even more irritated with him.

Praskovya: If you really are ill then you should get treatment! I insist that you go to see the eminent physician, Dr Leschititsky.

Narrator: He went, and everything was as he expected it to be. The waiting, the charade played out by the doctor – the tapping, the listening, the questions requiring futile replies, and the meaningful look which proclaimed, "Come, come sir, just rely on me and we'll sort it all out." All of this was familiar to Ivan. Just as he had put on a show in court for the man on trial, so the doctor put on a show for him.

Ivan Ilyich: Only one thing is important to me, Doctor. Is my condition dangerous or not?

Doctor Leschititsky: (*with an arrogant manner*) It is most probably that you are experiencing one of several maladies: a floating kidney, perhaps chronic catarrh, or a disease of the blind gut.

Narrator: For the doctor and quite probably for everyone, his illness didn't matter in the least, but for Ivan it was bad. He began to feel intense pity for himself and great bitterness against the doctor who was so indifferent to a question of such importance.

Ivan Ilyich: (*with disdain*) I imagine we sick people often ask you irrelevant questions. By and large, is it a dangerous illness or not?

Doctor Leschititsky: (*arrogantly*) I have already told you what I deem necessary and appropriate. Further evidence will come from the analyses.

Narrator: At home, in the middle of his account to his wife of his doctor's visit, his daughter Liza came in with her hat on, as she was about to go out with her mother. With an effort she sat down to listen to this tedious stuff. She could not contain herself for long, and her mother also stopped listening.

Praskovya: (*offhandedly*) Well, I'm delighted! Now mind you, take the medicine properly. We must leave now.

Ivan Ilyich: Well, who knows, perhaps it really is nothing much.

Narrator: Ivan became totally preoccupied with his illness and following the prescribed treatment. The pain grew no less, but he made great efforts to persuade himself that he felt better, and for a time he was able to deceive himself until something went wrong. Then he immediately felt the full force of the disease. He despaired.

Ivan Ilyich: (*raging*) I was just getting better, the medicine was finally beginning to work. These people are killing me. I need peace of mind. All this disruption infuriates me. The more I read the medical books and see the doctor, the worse I feel.

Narrator: He went to see several more specialists, but their diagnoses and advice only further confused Ivan and confirmed his doubts. He lost faith in all the physicians and fell into a state of profound gloom.

Ivan Ilyich: I mustn't give in to hypochondria. I must choose one doctor and keep strictly to his course of treatment. That's what I will do! Enough of this dithering.

Narrator: This was easy to say and impossible to do. The pain in his side seemed to grow steadily worse and was wearing him down. The taste in his mouth grew more peculiar, and his strength and appetite were both diminishing. He could no longer deceive himself. Something very significant was taking place inside him and he was the only one who knew about it. No one around him understood or cared. They thought that everything was going on as usual. That was what tormented Ivan more than anything.

His wife and daughter, who were caught up in their social whirl, were irritated by Ivan's demanding and cheerless manner.

Praskovya: You know, Ivan Ilyich, one day you take the drops and eat what you're ordered and go to bed in good time. The next day, if I don't keep an eye on you, you forget to take anything, you eat anything, and you stay up way too late at your card game.

Ivan Ilyich: What difference does that make? I can't sleep because of the pain.

Praskovya: What nonsense! You'll never get well like this. You'll just go on making us miserable. You are to blame for your illness, and this whole business is extremely unpleasant for me.

Narrator: Ivan believed that his co-workers had also developed a curious attitude toward him – as if he was soon to vacate his post. Even at his card games he became befuddled and his friends grew silent and gloomy. Ivan felt now as though poison permeated his whole existence and that he was poisoning the lives of others. With this knowledge and with his physical pain and his terror, Ivan spent most nights sleepless and then in the morning rose only to go through it all again. Every minute of every day was torment.

Ivan Ilyich: Why must I live in this way, on the very edge of destruction, without a single being who might understand and pity me?

Scene 3

Narrator: In mid-winter, Ivan's brother-in-law, Lacofsky, came to visit. Upon seeing Ivan for the first time, he opened his mouth to gasp and just stopped himself. That confirmed it all for Ivan.

Ivan Ilyich: What? Have I changed?

Lacofsky: Yes, there is a change.

Narrator: Later, Ivan Ilyich tiptoed up to Praskovya's closed sitting-room door and listened.

Praskovya: Nonsense, Lacofsky, you're exaggerating.

Lacofsky: What do you mean, exaggerating? You can't see it? He's a dead man, look at his eyes. There's no light in them. What's wrong with him, anyway?

Praskovya: No one knows. One of the doctors said one thing, but Leschititsky, the eminent doctor, said the opposite.

Narrator: Ivan Ilyich went into his study, lay down and began thinking. He remembered everything the doctors had told him. How the kidney had torn loose and was floating about. In his imagination he tried to catch his kidney and pin it down and stop it wandering. He decided to go and see Ivanovich's friend, Doctor Nikolayev, once again.

Doctor Nikolayev: There is some little thing, a minute little something, in the blind gut. It can all get better. It is just a matter of increasing the energy of one organ and diminishing the activity of another. Absorption will take place and everything will get better.

Narrator: Ivan went home and occupied his mind with work. The guests arrived and Ivan spent the evening in a cheerful manner. Later, he took his leave and went into the small room off his study where he had been sleeping since his illness had begun. He began thinking.

Ivan Ilyich: I can see how the correction of my blind gut can occur. Absorption is taking place, evacuation occurs, correct functioning is re-established. Yes, that's how it should be. We just have to give nature a hand. I just have to take my medicine steadily and avoid adverse influence. Already I feel a little better, a lot better. When I pinch my side it doesn't even hurt. It is really a lot better already. That blind gut is setting itself right, it is becoming absorbed.

Narrator: But suddenly he felt the familiar old, dull, gnawing pain and the familiar disgusting stuff in his mouth. His heart contracted, and his head clouded.

Ivan Ilyich: My God! My God! It will never end! It's not a matter of blind gut or the kidney but of life and . . . death. Yes, there was life and now it's going. It's going and I can't hold it back. Why should I deceive myself? It is obvious to everyone except me that I'm dying, and it's only a question of how many weeks, days even now, maybe.

I'll be no more and then what will there be? Nothing. Where will I be when I am no longer? Is this really death? Go away, I don't want you. Yes, death. And none of them knows and none of them wants to know and none of them is sorry. They're having fun. They don't care, but they'll die just like me. Idiocy! Sooner for me, later for them, but it will come. And they're happy. Mindless brutes!

I must calm down and think everything through from the beginning. There was the beginning of the illness. I knocked my side, but it was the same before and after. It ached a bit and then a bit more, and then there were doctors and then depression, dreariness, doctors again, and I kept coming closer and closer to the abyss. And here I am wasted away, no light in my eyes. This is death and I'm thinking about my gut. I'm thinking about putting my kidney right and this is death. Can this really be death?

Narrator: Panic overcame Ivan Ilyich and he lost his breath. Losing his temper he knocked over the bedside table. Then, in despair, he fell back expecting instant death. The guests were leaving when Praskovya heard something fall. She went to Ivan's room.

Praskovya: What's the matter?

Ivan Ilyich: Nothing. I knocked the table over by mistake.

Praskovya: You know, I think we should get Leschititsky to visit you here.

Narrator: Praskovya sat with Ivan a bit longer; then kissed him on the forehead. At that moment, he hated her with all the strength of his soul and had to make an effort not to push her away.

Praskovya: The last guests are leaving. I must go. Goodnight.

Scene 4

Narrator: In the depths of his soul Ivan knew that he was dying, but he could not get used to the idea and he could not accept it.

Ivan Ilyich: It cannot be right for me to die. That would be too terrible. If I had to die, I would have known it. My inner voice would have told me so. Now look! It can't be, but it is. How can it be? How can I understand it? I will find ways to take my mind from all this. I'll get back to work. After all, that was my life. I will forget this thinking about death.

Narrator: He went back to court, chatted with his friends and took his place on the bench as he always had done and opened the proceedings. But suddenly the pain in his side started its business, sucking away at him. *It* came up and stood right in front of him and looked at him and he froze. The light died out of his eyes.

Ivan Ilyich: Surely, *it* can't be the only truth? My court duties can no longer free me from *it. It* draws attention to itself. Regardless of what I do to forget, there *it* is, the same thing still crouching there, gnawing away. I can no longer forget, *it* is distinctly staring at me. What is the point of it all?

Narrator: Ivan went home and back to his study to lie down. He was alone with *it* again. Face to face with *it*, and nothing to do but look at *it* and grow cold.

Scene 5

Narrator: Imperceptibly, during the third month of Ivan Ilyich's illness, it happened that his wife, his daughter, the servants, his friends, his doctors and most of all he, himself, understood that their only interest was in how quickly he would die and free the living from the burden of his presence and himself from the suffering. Despite the use of opium and the increased injections of morphine, Ivan slept less and less and the pain increased more and more. But the need to take care of his excretions was the most unbearable. This situation tormented Ivan – the dirt, the indecency, the smell, and the knowledge that another person had to participate. But in his torment, his consolation came to light. It was Gerasim, the peasant who served at the table, who always came to carry out the soil. He was always bright and cheerful. At first Ivan was discomforted by him, but one day after Ivan was getting up from the commode, he was unable to pull up his trousers, and fell exhausted into a nearby armchair.

Ivan Ilyich: Gerasim.

Gerasim: Can I do anything for you?

Ivan Ilyich: Please help me. I think it must be unpleasant for you. You must forgive me. I can't help it.

Gerasim: Not at all, sir. Why shouldn't I take a little trouble? You're not well.

Narrator: Gerasim cheerfully removed the pan from the commode and left the room to dispose of it. When he returned a few moments later, Ivan was still in the armchair.

Ivan Ilyich: Gerasim, could you please help me again? Just lift me up. It's hard for me on my own even though I told others I could.

Gerasim: Of course. Let me just steady you as you stand, and then I can pull up your trousers.

Ivan Ilyich: Please take me over to the divan. How lightly and how well you do everything. Move that chair for me, please, under my legs and put the cushion under them. I feel better when my legs are high.

Narrator: Gerasim did these tasks carefully and with great kindness. It seemed to Ivan that when Gerasim was holding his legs high they felt best, and when placed lower on the cushion the pain returned.

Ivan Ilyich: Gerasim, are you busy at the moment?

Gerasim: Not in the least, your honor.

Ivan Ilyich: What have you still got to do?

Gerasim: There's only the wood to chop for tomorrow.

Ivan Ilyich: Then hold my legs up high, could you?

Gerasim: Of course I can.

Ilyich Ivan: But what about the firewood?

Gerasim: Don't worry about that, sir. I'll find time.

Narrator: Ivan Ilyich asked Gerasim to sit down and hold his legs, and talk to him. It all seemed to make him feel better while Gerasim was holding up his legs. From that time on, Ivan Ilyich began calling for him occasionally. Gerasim held his legs up willingly and talked to him with a lightness, simplicity and kindness that touched Ivan Ilyich. He was offended by healthy and good spirits in everyone else, but Gerasim's strength and cheerfulness soothed him rather than hurt him.

Ivan Ilyich suffered most of all from the lies – the lie that everyone accepted that he was just ill and not dying, that he only needed to keep calm and take his medicine and something good would happen. But he knew better. There would be only pain and agonizing death. And most of all, he resented that they forced him to participate in these lies. Somehow he could not find the courage to say to them, "Stop lying!"

Ivan Ilyich: Everyone around me reduces my death to a casual unpleasantness, an offense against the propriety that I have served all my life. No one pities me, because they don't understand my situation. Only Gerasim understands and is sorry for me. Gerasim knows that it is good for me when he holds my legs. And many times he holds my legs on his shoulders for an entire night and doesn't go to bed.

Gerasim: You mustn't worry, your honor. I'll get sleep another time. With thee so poorly, how couldn't I spare a little trouble? We'll all go someday, why not take a little trouble?

Narrator: After moments of great pain, Ivan wanted someone to pity him like a sick child would be pitied. And while he was ashamed at the thought, he longed to be stroked, kissed, cried over a little. In his relationship with Gerasim there was something like this, and consequently this relationship brought Ivan great comfort.

Scene 6

Narrator: One day as Ivan Ilyich washed his face, brushed his teeth and combed his hair, he became frightened by what he saw in the mirror. The look of his thin hair clinging to his pallid forehead was gruesome. He dared not look at the rest of his body. Beyond the pain, it was the misery of his existence that caused the most suffering for Ivan.

Just then the door bell rang and it was the doctor. Ivan, sensing who was at the door, made up his mind that he would tell the doctor that he couldn't go on like this and that he must think of something.

Narrator: The doctor breezed in, fresh, brisk, fat, and cheerful. He knew his expression was inappropriate here, but he had put it on once and for all and could not take it off again, like a man who had put on tails in the morning and driven off to pay a round of calls with no opportunity to change. As he approached Ivan, he rubbed his hands together briskly.

Doctor Leschititsky: My hands are chilly. It's quite a frost. Let me just get warm. Well now, how . . .

Ivan Ilyich: How did I pass the night?

Narrator: Ivan Ilyich looked at the doctor with an expression that asks "Will you never feel ashamed of your lies?" But the doctor did not want to understand his question.

Ivan Ilyich: It's all so dreadful. The pain won't stop, not even for a little. If only there was something.

Doctor Leschititsky: Yes, you sick men always say that. Well now, I think I've gotten a little warmer. How do you do today?

Narrator: As the doctor set a serious expression, he began to examine his patient, tapping and listening. Ivan Ilyich knew definitely that this was all nonsense, a hollow sham. But he allowed himself to be taken in, as in the old days when he gave in to the lawyers' speeches when he knew perfectly well that they were all lying and why they were lying.

Praskovya entered the room, moved to Ivan, and kissed him. Ivan Ilyich scrutinized her all over, taking exception to her plump, white, clean hands and neck, her shiny hair and bright eyes, full of life. He detested her with all the strength of his soul. And her touch made him suffer from his surge of hatred. Her attitude toward him and his illness was still the same. Just as the doctor had worked out an attitude toward his patients which he could no longer shake off, so she had worked out her attitude toward him – that he wasn't doing something he ought to be doing, and it was all his fault, while she lovingly reproached him.

Praskovya: He just won't do as he's told! He will not take the drops on time. But the main thing is, he lies down in a position that must surely be bad for him, with his legs in the air.

Doctor Leschititsky: What are we to do? These invalids sometimes think up the funniest things, but we can forgive them.

Narrator: With the exam completed, Praskovya announced that she had invited Mikhail Danilovich, an ordinary doctor, to visit while the distinguished doctor was there so that he could discuss Ivan's condition with him. Danilovich arrived at the appointed hour and once again there were the tappings and listenings and significant conversations about the kidney and blind gut in Ivan's presence and in the next room. All this nonsense, instead of the real question of life and death.

Doctor Leschititsky: Don't worry, Ivan Ilyich, we will pounce on these conditions this very minute and force them to behave.

Ivan Ilyich: (*timidly, yet hopeful*) Is there any chance of recovery?

Doctor Leschititsky: One cannot promise anything, but there is a possibility. Goodbye for now.

Scene 7

Narrator: Praskovya returned late that night and entered his room.

Praskovya: I think Gerasim should leave now. I would like to sit with you myself.

Ivan Ilyich: No. Go.

Praskovya: Are you suffering a lot?

Ivan Ilyich: It doesn't matter.

Praskovya: Take some opium.

Narrator: Ivan consented and drank it. She went away. Ivan was in an oppressive state of unconsciousness until three in the morning. It seemed to him that he and his pain were being pushed deeper and deeper into a long, narrow, black sack, yet couldn't be pushed right through. It was agonizing. He was afraid, yet wanted to fall through. He struggled against it, yet tried to help. Suddenly, he tore free and fell and came to. There he was, lying with his emaciated stockinged feet resting on Gerasim's shoulders. There was the same interminable pain.

Ivan Ilyich: You can go away, Gerasim.

Gerasim: It doesn't matter. I'll sit a while.

Ivan Ilyich: No, do go.

Narrator: Gerasim left and then, without constraint, Ivan cried like a child. He cried for his helplessness, his terrible loneliness, people's cruelty, God's cruelty, and the absence of God.

Ivan Ilyich: God, why have You done all this? Why did You bring me here? What have I done that You torment me so dreadfully? But I know You will not answer. Go on, batter me! But for what? What have I done to You? What is it for?

Narrator: Then Ivan stopped crying and grew quiet as though he were listening not to a voice speaking to him, but to the voice of his own soul.

Ivan Ilyich: You ask me what do I want? What do I need? Not to suffer. To live. Live how, you ask? Live like I did before. Pleasantly.

There was something good for me as a child, but that person is no more. Then in law school there was something genuinely good there – enjoyment, friendship, hopes. There were good moments in my Governor's service, and I remember love for women. As I think through my life, there is less and less good. My marriage – at first so happy, then disillusion. The hypocrisy, the anxieties about money all those 20 years.

So what is this? What is it for? Surely it can't be that my life was so pointless, so wrong? And if it was that wrong and that pointless, then why die and die in pain? Something's not right here.

Maybe I didn't live as I should. But how could that be, when I did everything as I should have done? I want to live as I lived in court. Here he comes, the judge. But I'm not to blame. What is my guilt? Why this misery?

Scene 8

Narrator: Two weeks passed and Ivan Ilyich did not rise from his divan, lying nearly all the time with his face to the wall. He suffered alone. From the beginning of his illness, his life seemed split into two opposing and alternating moods – either despair and the expectation of incomprehensible and terrible death, or hope and the absorbing scrutiny of his bodily functions – his kidney or his gut. He existed now in a loneliness which could not have been more complete.

Ivan Ilyich: Just as my suffering grows worse and worse now, so the whole of my life went worse and worse. If only I could understand what it is for. It could only be explained if one could say I hadn't lived as I should. But to accept that would be quite impossible. There is no explanation! Suffering. Death. For what?

160

Narrator: The next two weeks passed in this way. One day, Petrishev, Liza's fiancé, made a formal proposal to marry Ivan's daughter. That same night, Ivan suffered another change for the worse. When Praskovya and his daughter, Liza, went into his room to tell him about the proposal, Ivan was moaning and staring fixedly in front of him. Praskovya started talking about medicines. But she stopped suddenly when he shifted his gaze to her and she saw the terrible look of hatred he had for her.

Ivan Ilyich: For the love of Christ, let me die in peace! You will both soon be free of me.

Narrator: Both women fell silent, sat a while, and then left the room.

Liza: (*whining*) It's just as though we were doing it *to* him! I'm sorry for Papa, but why should we be made miserable?

Narrator: Doctor Nikolayev arrived soon, and Ivan answered his tiresome questions.

Ivan Ilyich: You know perfectly well you can do nothing, so leave it alone. You cannot even alleviate my suffering. Leave it!

Narrator: The doctor left the room and informed Praskovya that things were very bad and only opium could relieve the pain.

Doctor Nikolayev: His physical suffering is intense, but his spiritual suffering is worse, and that is what torments him most of all.

Narrator: Ivan's spiritual suffering had come suddenly during the night as he looked at Gerasim's kind, sleepy face with its high cheekbones. It was then that Ivan questioned his life.

Ivan Ilyich: What if in reality the whole of my life was not done right? Could it be true that I have lived my whole life not as I should have done? It occurs to me that I never did fight against what people in high positions deemed good when they were wrong . . . I shrugged it off. And my work and the construction of my life and my family and my social and professional interests – all of them might be not the right thing. And if this is so, and I am leaving life in the knowledge that I have ruined everything that was given to me and it can't be put right, then what? All of my life was not the right thing, all of it was a dreadful, vast lie.

Praskovya: Ivan, sweetest, take communion, do this for me. It can't do any harm and it often helps.

Ivan Ilyich: What? Take communion? What for? There's no need. And yet . . .

Praskovya: I'll send for our priest, he's so nice.

Narrator: When the priest heard his confession, Ivan felt a kind of ease from his doubts and his suffering and a moment's hope came to him. He started thinking again about his blind gut and the possibility of putting it right. He took the sacrament with tears in his eyes. His hope of life rose again.

Ivan Ilyich: To live, I want to live!

Praskovya: It's true, isn't it? You're better.

Ivan Ilyich: Yes.

Narrator: As he looked at Praskovya – her clothes, the way she was put together, the expression on her face, the sound of her voice – it all said one thing to him. It was true – everything he had once lived by was a lie. And as soon as he thought that, the suffering returned, and with it the knowledge of inevitable, imminent death.

Ivan Ilyich: Go away! Get out! Let me be!

Scene 9

Narrator: From that minute began the three days of unremitted screaming, so dreadful it could be heard with horror beyond two closed doors.

Ivan Ilyich: I am lost. There is no return. The end has come, the very end. No!!!

I am being thrust into the black hole. I am unable to crawl into it for myself. It is because my life has been bad, that is the reason I cannot crawl into the hole. Let me go! Let me get into the hole, do not hold me tight. Why do you torment me?

Narrator: On the third day, an hour before Ivan's death, his little son, Vassili, crept into his father's room and came up to his bed. The dying man was still screaming desperately and throwing his arms about. His hand fell on Vassili's head. The boy caught hold of it, pressed it to his lips and burst into tears.

It was just at this point that Ivan Ilyich fell through the hole. He saw the glimmer of light and it became clear to him that his life had not been what it should have been, but that it could still be put right.

Ivan Ilyich: What is it I feel? Someone is kissing my hand.

Narrator: He opened his eyes and looked at his son. He wife came into the room and he glanced at her. She was gazing at him with a look of despair, her mouth open, tears on her nose and cheeks. He felt sorry for her. Too weak to speak, Ivan thought, "Yes, I am making them miserable. They're sorry for me, but it will be better for them when I'm dead."

Ivan Ilyich: Take my son out. Sorry for him. Sorry for you. . . . Propusti.

Narrator: He had wanted to say "prosti" – forgive me. But he said "propusti" – let me pass. Lacking the strength to correct himself, he gave up, knowing that the one who needed to know would understand him. Suddenly it became clear that what had been tormenting him was suddenly leaving him, falling away on all sides. He was sorry for them, he had to free them and free himself from all this pain.

Ivan Ilyich: How good and how simple. And where has the pain gone? Come on, where are you, pain? Yes, there it is. Well, never mind, let it be. And death? Where is it? But where is my fear of death? I cannot find it. There is no death. Instead of death there is only light! What joy!!

Narrator: For him it all happened in a moment. For those around him, his agony continued for two hours. Gradually the snoring gurgle came less frequently.
  "It is finished", someone above him said.

Ivan Ilyich: Death is finished. There is no more death.

Narrator: He drew the air into himself, stopped in mid breath, stretched and died.

DISCUSSION QUESTIONS

Below is an example of the types of questions that are used to engage participants following a readers' theater.

1 What is the time span of the play? In what era does it take place?
2 How would you describe the overall tenor, style, and language of the story?
3 What is the plot (the action, and the ordering of events into meaning)?
4 From what perspective is the story told? Is the author trying to convey a message? If so, what is it? What does the story leave out?
5 Who is the narrator? Describe the narrator's position/demeanor from the beginning to the end. Is the narrator reliable?
6 What were some of your feelings as you read through the story?
7 How do members of Ivan's family relate to his illness? What are your feelings about the following characters: Ivan, Ivan's colleagues, Praskovya, Ivan's son Vassili, Ivan's daughter Liza, Gerasim, the physicians?

8   What does the author mean by the "black sack of darkness"?

9   Who in the story needs to be cared for? Who is the primary caregiver and what is the role of this individual in Ivan's life?

10 How would you care for Ivan? What might you carry from this play into your own caregiving?

11 What do you think about the ending of the story?

12 Do you think Tolstoy's existential concerns and his fear of death influenced his writing? If so, how?

13 Write one or two questions that you would ask about the play.

PART 3

Narrative Competence and Its Outcomes

Clusters of new and/or neglected skills are required to live and practice narratively in current health care environments. A new narrative competence in conjunction with scientific competence is required for an effective and fulfilling practice of health care. Each of six narrative skills is examined in Chapter 6, and the application of these skills to clinical encounters is highlighted. Readers have the opportunity to practice some of these skills through a set of narrative stretching exercises. Chapter 7 discusses the evidence for narrative success and risks of non-narrative practice.

CHAPTER 6

Skills for the Practice of Narrative Medicine

> Patients have suffered long enough the consequences of a medicine practiced by doctors without these skills – doctors who cannot follow a narrative thread; who cannot adopt an alien perspective; who become unreliable narrators of other people's stories; who are deaf to voice and images; and who do not always include in their regard human motives, yearnings, symbols, and the fellowship born of a common language.
>
> **Rita Charon (1: 29)**

cont.

- WRITING REFLECTIVELY AND TELLING COMPLEX CLINICAL STORIES
  - Writing Reflectively
  - Listening to and Telling Stories in a Group
- REASONING WITH STORIES
- ENGAGING IN NARRATIVE ETHICS
- A TRANSFORMATION

KEY IDEAS

- The practice of mindfulness teaches caregivers to be present and listen mindfully.
- Moral imagination enables the clinician to bear witness to a patient's life experience, strengthens her empathic capacities, and lays the groundwork for shared patient–clinician roles.
- Practicing the skills of close reading and analysis of literary work teaches practitioners to interact more fully with the complexities of their patients' illnesses.
- Writing reflectively and telling clinical stories enable practitioners to become more reflective about their own personal and professional lives and development.
- Listening to and telling clinical stories improve practitioners' abilities to understand and interpret their own experiences, clarify their values and beliefs, and form their professional identities.
- Reading, discussing, and telling stories that present moral issues develop practitioners' skills in making sound ethical decisions.

WHY FOCUS ON NARRATIVE SKILLS?

Narrative skills that we observe among medical professionals are highly variable. At one end of the spectrum are practitioners who seem naturally gifted with skills that enable them to provide compassionate care and to develop satisfying and healing relationships with patients. By contrast, at the other end are those whom Charon identifies above, who sorely lack these critical skills, and whom patients describe as indifferent, uncaring, or cold. Many have lost skills to burgeoning scientific technology, high patient volume, sub-specialization, or pressing economic considerations. Some perhaps failed to develop effective skills in their professional training, and others seem to be unaware of the importance of these skills. The result is that:

- the patient may not tell the whole story
- the patient may not ask the most troubling questions
- the patient may not feel that she has been heard
- the diagnostic workup may be unfocused and faulty

- clinical care may be marked by "non-compliance"
- a therapeutic relationship may not develop
- the clinician may feel professionally dissatisfied.

The narratively competent clinician possesses the wisdom to know when and with whom to pursue deep connection.

How do we improve upon this situation? A narrative-competence approach to illness, described by Greenhalgh (2: 28):

- views the illness, and the patient's efforts to deal with it, as an unfolding story within his or her wider lifeworld
- acknowledges the patient as the narrator of the story and as the subject (rather than the object) of the tale, and hence gives central importance to the patient's own role in defining, managing, and making sense of the illness
- recognizes that a single problem or experience will generate multiple interpretations, and that the key version to be addressed is the one framed and developed by the patient
- embraces both trust (the patient makes herself vulnerable and stakes confidence in the clinician in the act of telling her story) and obligation (the clinician incurs ethical duties in the act of hearing it)
- views the spoken (and enacted) dialogue between health professional and patient as an integral part of the clinical management.

Narrative competence is much more than the sum of its parts. We see it as the way in which medical professionals, in collaboration with their patients, distinguish the relevant from the irrelevant and clarify perception, intent, and meaning. Together with the patient, the practitioner co-constructs and interprets her illness story, integrating the presenting disease or particular condition with the effect that it has on the frame and scope of her entire life. We recall here Bruner's discussion (*see* Chapter 4) of the two distinct landscapes that all stories construct – an *action* landscape and a *consciousness* landscape, where we learn what the individuals of the story think and feel. It is here in these two landscapes – in the understanding, reconstructing, and moving forward – that the critical relationship between the patient and the caregiver unfolds.

How can health care professionals whose narrative skills are minimal, lie dormant, or have atrophied over time, improve their capabilities? Can the skills be learned in the same way that technical skills and medical knowledge are learned? We, along with others (3–5), believe that narrative training is the answer. Charon comments (4: 2):

> Narrative medicine brings a useful set of skills, tools, and perspectives to all doctors. Not only does it propose an ideal of medical care – attentive, attuned, reflective, altruistic, loyal, able to witness others' suffering and honor their narratives – that can inspire us all to better

medicine, [but] it also donates the methods by which to grow toward those ideals. Any doctor and any medical student can improve his capacity for empathy, reflection, and professionalism through serious narrative training.

In Chapter 3 we explored aspects of Stacey's theory of complex responsive processes of relating (CRPR), which we believe provides a theoretical understanding for the concept of relationship that is at the core of relationship-centered care. Furthermore, we argued that the meaning of relationship is narrative in character, and consequently the theory and practice of narrative medicine connects with the theory and practice of relationship-centered care. We maintain that narrative competence provides the practical means for enacting relationship-centered care. In this chapter we shall examine six narrative skills:

- practicing compassionate presence and mindful listening
- exercising moral imagination and practicing empathy
- reading and interpreting complex texts
- writing reflectively and telling complex clinical stories
- reasoning with stories
- engaging in narrative ethics.

We provide a rationale for each of the six skills, and describe our own teaching and learning experience with each of them. Although other skills could be added, the six narrative skills that we introduce are critical in that they logically and practically flow from Stacey's theory of complex responsive processes of relating, and serve as foundational elements for relationship-centered care.

The skills in question are not mutually exclusive. Rather, there is considerable overlap and interdependence among them. Two complex skills in particular lie at the very core of all the skills because they set the stage for interaction and understanding. The first of these is *practicing compassionate presence and mindful listening*. Recalling Dr Gardner's conversation with Mrs Flowers (*see* Chapter 3), clearly he could not have promptly cued in to her mention of pickle juice if he had not been attending closely and listening mindfully. The other central skill – *exercising moral imagination and practicing empathy* – enables an individual to imagine the lived experience of another and to determine the accuracy of that representation. Dr Gardner, in exercising his moral imagination, suspects that Mrs Flowers' mother has influence in the family and may be insistent upon her remedy. He probes this imaginative representation when he suggests that her mother could be present for the discussion of the pickle juice remedy. We envision these two skills as the force which gives agency to the others.

Because of the interconnectedness of the skills, educational techniques such as reading literature, telling and listening to stories, and analyzing poetry, other art forms, and stories depicted in movies can be used to stimulate the identification and development of the different narrative skills. In the Preface we noted that all four of us are educators from separate but related disciplines, with varied experience across all levels of medical education. The narrative exercises that we describe throughout this chapter and the many examples of reflective writing that we include have been drawn from the courses, seminars, and conferences we have conducted over the years, and from others that we have attended.

PRACTICING COMPASSIONATE PRESENCE AND MINDFUL LISTENING

When a person is struck by serious physical or psychological illness, the fear and anguish that often arise can be overwhelming. Will I die? How can I complete my work? What will become of my loved ones? Why is God punishing me? All of these are issues of the spirit. All reflect the felt discontinuities in the person's narrative identity – disruption in the coherence of the person's life story – concepts which we explored in Chapter 2 through the work of Brody, Carr, Linde, Rimmon-Kenan, and others. Narrative is the doorway to the spirit. Attending to the existential concerns of the patient will most likely result in a rich narrative exchange.

Compassionate Presence

One of the greatest gifts in a time of illness is to be attended by a practitioner who is technically competent, caring, and compassionate – one who can work to illuminate the meaning of the illness experience and help the patient to gain a renewed sense of hope for the return of wholeness and life continuity. Unfortunately, in today's fast-paced health care environment the patient may not always find such an individual. All too often patients meet caregivers who seem too harried to be totally present for them, and who appear unable or unwilling to engage in their stories. Patients may resent the lack of interconnection and may even begin to doubt the practitioner's competence. At other times, although the clinician appears to be present and caring, her lack of authenticity is immediately clear. It is quickly perceived that she is not really hearing or responding appropriately. On this matter Connelly writes (6: 420):

> In medical encounters as in social encounters, one person may feel abandoned or neglected when the other is not paying attention. . . . Patients may choose not to disclose symptoms or significant life events in the absence of confidence, support, and trust. . . . Being in the present moment involves time and awareness. Time is the present; it is now. It is not the future of the unknowable next moment; it is not the past with memories beginning to vanish. It is now. Awareness is conscious and personal; it is wakefulness and mindfulness of the happening of the moment; it involves thoughts, ideas, images, emotions, sensations, and movements.

The act of being mindfully present for a suffering patient is the tender core of the following story:

My friend suffers from chronic polymyositis and rheumatoid arthritis, each in its own right a severely debilitating disease. Surgery performed on her crooked and misshapen fingers has improved her hand capabilities somewhat, but the severe weakness of her muscles, along with the deformities of her feet, cause her to creep along slowly in baby steps, and even sitting can be torturous. Recently I drove her to the rheumatologist's office. When she emerged from the office and we returned to the car she was all smiles and exclaimed, "Dr Max is so wonderful. I am so blessed to have found both him and my sweetheart orthopedic guy."

"That's quite a testimonial", I said. Why are you so blessed? What's so great about them?" I asked.

"Every time I go to see Dr Max", she replied, "he sits right down in front of me and looks right into my eyes and asks me how I'm doing, and then explains what he thinks is going on and suggests what might help if I am willing. He always asks me if I understand, and he answers all my questions. Today, when I stood up to leave, he saw me inching along the wall for balance and he put his arm around my waist and took my hand and walked with me out to the lobby. Isn't he something? And you know, Dr Jake, my orthopedic surgeon, is just the same way. They're both so different from that first bozo doctor I had – he always made me feel like just another nobody. He was always in a hurry, he never sat down with me and he never listened to me. He just always told me what he was going to do about this and that, he wrote in his chart and then left the room.

Yes, I am truly blessed. Today I told Dr Max that I know I won't live very much longer and I wanted to thank him for all he has done for me and for being so kind and caring through all this. Tears came into his eyes – and mine, too."

LLP

Presence is paradoxical. It is part of being human, yet it is a skilled activity that must be consciously practiced. When mastered, it is an exceedingly effective way of relating to a patient's experience. As Connelly notes above, presence means being with the other person in this moment – physically, emotionally, and spiritually. It means being aware of one's own concerns, beliefs, and moral standards, yet not allowing them to confuse what's going on in the moment. It means being respectful of what the other is relating, and bearing empathic witness to her suffering, her fear, or her joy. Presence means connecting with the spirit of the other person and responding supportively – perhaps with a gesture or just with attentive silence. Presence is the grounding process of all the important elements of compassion and healing; it is the cornerstone of the therapeutic relationship (6–9). Presence is palpable. And perhaps it is most obvious when it is absent.

> There is a channel between voice and presence,
> a way where information flows.
> In disciplined silence the channel opens,
> with wandering talk, it closes.

Rumi (10: 25)

According to Rinpoche, a Tibetan Lama, and Shlim, an American physician (11), being mindfully present in the medical encounter demonstrates caring for the patient, and this kind of attentiveness results in fewer errors in medical judgment and inspires patients' confidence in the caregiver. Thus the mindful and compassionate practitioner functions more effectively and intelligently. Speaking about the importance of mindfulness, Ronald Epstein, a family physician, writes (8: 835): "The goals of mindful practice are to become more aware of one's own mental processes, listen more attentively, become flexible, recognize bias and judgment, and thereby act with principles and compassion." Launer (5) sees the mindful caregiver as an "observer–participant" who is able to co-construct a new story with the patient while at the same time observing and tracking its progress. This is a complex task that is explained in the following way by two spiritual leaders, Ram Das and Gorman (12: 119):

> The consciousness we have access to is greater than the particular thoughts we're having or skills we've mastered. We have all these. But we have perspectives as well – all within our spacious awareness. What's critical is that this awareness allows us to hear, along with everything else, whatever it is. The quiet mind makes possible an overall awareness of the total situation, including ourselves.

To better envision the mindful and compassionate practitioner, it is useful to consider how caregivers function with the number and variety of patients whom they meet daily. Patients who listen closely to the counsel we offer and who respond appropriately, and who are cooperative and compliant, are easy to work with. These are the ideal patients, and we feel good about caring for them. But what about the very different and difficult patients – those who are unhappy, ungrateful, irritable, abusive, and who never seem to change regardless of how much time we spend with them? How do we react to them? And then there is the patient who is weak, ineffective, and whiny – a "victim personality." In each situation, we must remember that here is an individual who is suffering spiritually, one who deserves our mindful and compassionate presence. How do we stay connected with her? How do we respond? Levinson describes a method that she terms *mining for gold* which she uses to change her feelings about a difficult patient. She learns something new about the patient (children, hobbies, common interests, etc.), and continues this focus throughout subsequent visits. Over time she reports that the relationship changes dramatically (13). The patient is more satisfied, makes fewer visits, accepts treatment more readily, and is more compliant.

Rinpoche and Shlim (11) remind us that dealing with a difficult patient is a special opportunity to display compassion and empathy. But how do we do this when we ourselves are provoked to anger and resentment by their behavior? It is precisely in these moments when we must stop, take a few deep breaths, and pull hard on our own spiritual bootstraps, knowing that without adequate tolerance and patience we cannot possibly be compassionate and empathic. Is it always possible to exercise such restraint? In order to prevent our own emotional upheaval and burnout we must be wise in setting limits and boundaries to the extent of our tolerance, and step back and re-establish equilibrium. We must learn to practice altruism conditioned by phronesis as discussed in Chapter 4.

Mindful Listening

In the outpatient office or at the hospital bedside, body language, non-intrusive body positioning, eye contact, and mindful listening are unmistakable indicators of presence. Most of us, in our professional education, learned how the first three of these skills affect our communication with others. However, fewer of us were taught or learned how to listen mindfully. Shafir posits that mindful listening is a key component of the therapeutic relationship (14: 13):

> Our goal in becoming mindful listeners is to quiet the internal noise to allow the whole message and the messenger to be understood. In addition, when we listen mindfully to others we help quiet down *their* internal noise. *When they notice that we are totally with them, people feel freer to cut out the layers of pretense to say what's really on their minds.* (emphasis added)

Mindful listening requires a lot of us. It requires a *desire* to listen, and it requires a quiet mind and concentration. And depending on the story we hear, it may cause us to feel some discomfort. Recognizing our discomfort, we must ask, "Do I have a moral obligation to attend to the matter in some way? Should I help my patient find meaning in this situation? How far should I go? How might it help my patient if I pursue this issue?" Regardless of what is happening around us, there are times when we choose to listen, and there are certain people to whom we choose to listen. Then there are situations when we *allow* distractions to interfere with our listening. In the medical encounter, distractions are ubiquitous and take many forms – pagers, office and hospital noise, time constraints, personal biases or prejudices, the offensive odors or attitudes of our patients, our own issues with status and power, the personal stressors of our own lives, and the focus that we give to the diagnosis and treatment of a disease, rather than to the story that our patient is relating to us.

Listen, if you can stand to.
Union with this Friend means not being who you've been
being instead silence: A place: A view
where language is inside seeing.

Rumi (10: 31)

Practice in quieting the mind is essential to eliminate the many distractions that intrude on our patient encounters. This requires that we practice a quieting activity daily until we are able to drop into our "quiet place" whenever we choose, and remain there for as long as necessary. A simple first step to becoming more peaceful and mindful is to repeat a brief mindfulness exercise every time we are about to enter the consultation or hospital room. Eventually it can become a useful habit.

One-Minute Mindfulness Exercise

First peruse the patient chart carefully in your usual manner and make note of the pertinent items that you feel are important for today's meeting. Next, stop altogether. Breathe deeply with your diaphragm and let the air out slowly. Relax and feel the floor beneath your feet supporting you. Become present to yourself – the concerns and emotions that you are feeling, your muscle tightness, your breathing and heart rate. Take several deep, slow breaths and release any feelings and tension you feel. Go into the center of yourself and let go of the many thoughts that may be racing around in your head. Knock and enter the room, consciously open and ready for whatever you might hear or experience with this patient.

LLP

By observing our own mind over a period of time, we realize that the mind is not always racing and chaotic. There are times when it seems almost blank, and there are other times when it is sharp, focused, and clear. When we are with patients we need to have a quiet mind and feel peaceful, and yet at the same time be alert, open, receptive, and able to concentrate fully. These capacities can be cultivated through the practice of meditation. Simultaneously, we benefit from the increased relaxation and reduced stress that meditation provides. Jon Kabat-Zinn, a leader in the field of mind–body medicine, speaks about the practice of meditation (15: 21, 61):

> Until recently the very word *meditation* tended to evoke raised eyebrows and thoughts about mysticism and hocus-pocus in many people. In part that was because people did not understand that meditation is really about paying attention. . . . And since paying attention is something that everybody does, at least occasionally, meditation is not as foreign or irrelevant to our life experience as we might have thought. . . . Meditation is . . . "falling awake, not falling into a trance." . . . We call

the heart of the formal meditation practice "sitting meditation" or simple "sitting." As with breathing, sitting is not foreign to anyone. We all sit, nothing special about that. But mindful sitting is different from ordinary sitting in the same way that mindful breathing is different from ordinary breathing. The difference, of course, is your awareness.

There is nothing magical or mystical about meditation. It is simply a method of using the breath to quiet the mind and let go of intrusive thoughts. Meditation is easily learned (see the Further Activities section at the end of this chapter for helpful sources). Practice in meditation should begin by finding a quiet location where there are no distractions and where you can sit in a comfortable position on the floor or on a chair. Rest your arms on the chair arms or place them comfortably in your lap or on top of your thighs. Sit with your head, neck, and back aligned vertically but not rigid – "sitting with dignity" as it is termed by Kabat-Zinn (15).

Sitting Exercise

The simplest way to begin learning to meditate is to use the breath as an anchor for your mind. Close your eyes to shut out the outside world and relax, allowing yourself to feel the chair (or the floor) supporting you. Notice the breath gently passing in and out of your nose. Don't try to control or think about how you are breathing, just notice how very natural and relaxed it is. Feel your abdomen rising and falling. Feel the moment of absolute peace between your breaths. Try to go into the center of your being. When thoughts come, give respect to them, let them go, and immediately return to your peaceful breathing. There will be times when suddenly a particular feeling arises – maybe sadness, anger, fear, etc. Do not try to bury it. Recognize it, understand it, honor it, then let go of it and return to your breathing. Repeat this sitting practice throughout your day whenever you can, even if it is only for a few moments at a time. It is important to vary the length of your sitting practice so that you begin to understand how deeply engaged you can become and how you can gain the most benefit.

LLP

The goal is to be able to arrive at this peaceful place easily and often during your busy day. Once you become comfortable with this simple and gentle sitting meditation, you can begin to add mindfulness to your practice in small increments in the following way.

Mindfulness Meditation Exercise

Begin with the sitting practice. When you get comfortable and centered in your quiet space, bring into your consciousness one feeling you get from the room – the warmth or coolness, an air movement, an odor, the nature of the room. Just allow this one feeling into your consciousness, and still pay attention to your breathing. When other thoughts enter your mind, just let them go and focus again on your breathing and the feeling you have chosen from the room. The next time you practice, add a different feeling from the room. Another time while you are sitting, focus on a place of tension or discomfort in your body, but remember to continue with the gentle natural conscious breathing. Breathe into the place of discomfort or tension and feel it ease. Finally, you can focus on one of your own thoughts, a worry or problem, along with your breathing – how you feel about that thought, what it does in your body, what you would like to do about the problem. Always pay attention to your natural and easy breathing.

LLP

The eventual goal of mindful meditation is to maintain a quiet mind, yet be totally mindful of your surroundings, your body, and your own thoughts. In your medical practice, you need to be mindful of the story that your patient is relating to you. Other ways to quiet the mind include focusing on your natural and gentle breath while repeating a mantra or listening to music, while watching rustling leaves or lapping waves, or while enjoying a sunset. Yoga, Tai Chi, and slow meditative walking are effective forms of moving meditation. The very best time for meditation practice is upon arising in the morning. However, you might find another part of the day that better suits your lifestyle. Being skillful at meditation enables the health care practitioner to enter a state of being fully present and attending to the patient.

Finally, we should note that research on the meditation process shows that it has profound health benefits for both patients and practitioners.[*] It has been found that a 10-minute meditation each morning is an effective way to maintain a healthy blood pressure. For clinicians, a regular practice of meditation effectively reduces stress, promotes emotional steadiness, and prevents burnout.

EXERCISING MORAL IMAGINATION AND PRACTICING EMPATHY

Humans are unable to exist comfortably with the many broken and discontinuous scenes and happenings of their lives (22). By telling stories, we attempt to unify these disparate entities in order to better understand and assign reason for our experiences. Through stories we identify and interpret ourselves, examine our commitments, improve our lives, and find meaning and purpose in our existence. Telling stories is our way of creating coherence in our lives – it is a basic element of what it means to be human. Stories sustain us and help us to

---

[*] Research indicates that meditation effectively reduces symptoms commonly associated with anxiety and stress (16), it lowers mood disturbances and stress symptoms in cancer patients (17), it reduces stress in hypertensive patients and in patients with carotid atherosclerosis (18, 19), it improves coping in patients with chronic pain (20), it enhances health-related quality of life, and it reduces physical symptoms and psychological stress (21).

endure our lifeworlds. We find ways to associate current situations with our past and look outward to the future. As we interact with patients around their lived experiences, we relate to the patterns in our patients' stories as they attempt to organize symptoms, causes, concerns, and life issues in ways that might explain their current circumstances. In Stacey's terms, these are "narrative in its making" and *intrinsically non-linear – complex patterns that shift unpredictably and amplify small differences in understanding.* As practitioners we work with patients to seek unifying themes and re-emplot their often fragmented stories into more coherent and more stable narratives, recognizing that illness stories evolve over time and are neither permanent nor determined. We do this by exercising our moral imagination – our ethical sensitivity – an action aptly described by Stacey as a complex collaborative process which brings coherence and order to patients' narratives (*see* Chapter 3).

The Character of Moral Imagination

The act of co-authoring new narratives with our patients demands *moral imagination*. This in turn gives rise to an increase in our capacity for empathy. In Chapter 4 we discussed various constructs of moral imagination, and defined moral imagination as including the commitments to:

1 understand one's own values, biases, viewpoints, and brokenness as the meaningful substrate that one brings to the caregiving relationship
2 remain open to the particularity and meaning of a patient's experience, and to attend to them mindfully
3 seek to understand the patient's lived experience, and operate in the narrative of that lived experience
4 seek within that narrative to co-construct a new narrative aimed at healing.

An essential skill underlying commitments 2 and 3 in particular is the ability to *bear witness* to the suffering or joy of the patient by attending closely, listening mindfully, remaining connected yet objective, and interacting sensitively. This ability has been labeled *vicarious imagination* (5), *empathic witnessing* (23), and *witnessing imagination* (24). Regardless of how it is termed, the skill requires concentrated effort and practice. The practitioner imaginatively puts herself in the patient's position, projects herself into their lifeworld, and lives out the story as it is being told (4, 24–26). Inside this "other world" she observes, knows, and connects with all that she finds there – pain and suffering, anger, worry and fear, and healing and joy. She begins to comprehend what the patient is experiencing.

There are many training techniques that can be employed to stimulate the moral imagination of medical professionals and students, such as:

- the use of narrative worlds effectively depicted in literature, poetry, or plays
- personal experiences in patient care
- artwork, film, or other images
- individual or group patient interviews.

In general, our exercises have three parts. The trainee is first asked to imaginatively enter the lifeworld of a patient (or a character in another story). Next, we ask them to write reflectively, and finally we ask them to share and discuss their stories with the group. We noted at the outset of this chapter that the six narrative skills overlap and complement one another. Consequently, exercises that we describe later are also useful here for developing the skills of exercising moral imagination and expressing clinical empathy. It is our hope that the examples of exercises we illustrate will trigger the creative bent of our readers to devise other meaningful techniques.

Developing Moral Imagination Using Readers' Theater and Film

When combined with the task of writing from a character's perspective about an issue, readers' theater* is a useful exercise for enabling participants to stretch their moral imagination. We adapted Tolstoy's *The Death of Ivan Ilyich* into a play to provide you with an at-hand example of medical readers' theater (*see* Interlude on page 149). Leo Tolstoy, who lived and wrote in mid-nineteenth-century Russia, suffered existential anguish and a fear of death which considerably influenced his writing. Eventually his fears and spiritual concerns resulted in his conversion to a Buddhist/Christian belief system. *The Death of Ivan Ilyich*, which was published in 1886, is a vivid portrayal of suffering and death.

For many years right up until his death, Ivan Ilyich pursued social status through a successful and satisfying professional life as a magistrate of the courts. However, his personal life was sorely marred by a miserably disruptive marriage. In his last days of life, Ivan found himself surrounded by arrogant and disingenuous physicians, a disagreeable family who openly displayed disdain for his suffering, and colleagues who now thought only of their own career advancements upon Ivan's death. The only person who provides unconditional caring is the house servant, Gerasim. Only with death's release did Ivan find peace and redemption.

The emotions triggered in the listeners and in the readers by performing any readers' theater, particularly those which are rife with emotional undertones, are usually quite obvious during the reading. At the conclusion of the performance, participants are asked for specific and detailed reactions to the overall story, the characters within the story, and the attitudes of the main characters. Next, participants are requested to choose one character for their reflective writing, to imagine that character's situation from his or her viewpoint, and then write in the voice of that character. Consistently, we see in participants' reflective pieces the strong imaginative ability of each of the writers to enter into the experiences of their chosen character and to capture the emotions and concerns that they find there.

---

* A readers' theater is a play in which the actors, rather than memorizing and performing lines, read the lines directly from the text. A useful collection of plays in this format can be found in Savitt TL, editor. *Medical Readers' Theater: a guide and scripts.* Iowa City, IA: University of Iowa Press; 2002.

The same strategy of using creative writing can be connected with the use of film. In our seminars we have used a video entitled *A Choice for K'aila* (27), which documents the dilemma of a native Canadian couple who are urged by their pediatrician to accept a liver transplant for their ailing baby boy, K'aila. Based on their cultural beliefs, and also fearing the possibility of great suffering and perhaps even death of their child at a later time, the parents refuse the transplant. The physician, feeling strongly that transplantation is the appropriate medical choice, refers the case to the social service agency, which propels it into the legal system. To avoid court proceedings, the family leaves its home and moves into another Province. After an extended legal process, the court finds in favor of the family. Meanwhile the baby, K'aila, has died peacefully in the arms of his family.

After viewing the film, participants are asked to select a character and in that person's voice to write about their situation. The following pieces were written by two resident physicians as they imagined the feelings of K'aila's father. In the first piece, we share in the anguish that the father feels as he is summoned home to be with his dying son. In the second piece, the writer explores the scorn that the father might feel for the doctor and his medical decisions.

> I think I have been waiting for this summons my entire life. Everything up until now has simply been leading up to this moment. What will come after I cannot even begin to imagine. Part of me wishes for oblivion. My heart is racing, but the air is still. My breath cascades painfully into my lungs, and my bones feel brittle. My footsteps are the loneliest sound I have ever heard. I barely steady my trembling hands as I move toward my home, my wife who awaits my presence, and my dying son.
>
> *Raafia Mir*

> Sure, I asked this doctor for advice on how best to help my son, but it seems as if he is so preoccupied with being a hero and winning in his daily battles of life and death that he has lost sight of my child as a living, breathing human being with thoughts, feelings, preferences, and beliefs. Of course I want all that can be done for my son, but that doesn't mean going beyond what God has already determined for him. What is worse is that this doctor wants to desecrate another person's body and to involve my son in the process. I wonder if I made a mistake in consulting him . . .
>
> *Anonymous*

We see in these reflective pieces the strong imaginative ability of the writers to enter into the experience of the father and to capture the emotions that they envision existing there. We anticipate that the value of this exercise will come later when perhaps these physicians encounter similar situations with their patients and are better prepared to engage meaningfully in the patients' concerns.

Developing Moral Imagination Using Photographs

This exercise uses a series of photographic portraits to challenge trainees' power of imagination. We display each photograph for about 30 seconds, and ask participants to choose one of the individuals to imagine as their patient. The individuals in the photos vary in age, physical characteristics, race, environment, and emotional expression. Then we ask the participants to write imaginatively about that person's story and how they, the practitioner, might interact with that "patient." They are encouraged to write in the voice of the patient.

The photograph chosen by a first-year medical student depicted an obese man wearing baggy trousers and a rumpled shirt and sweater, standing on a scale, probably in a doctor's office.

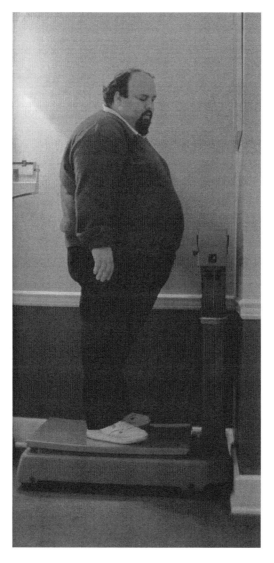

The young trainee wrote a poignant and emotional narrative entitled *What We Are.*

What We Are

I giggle from my windowsill
who's the funny fat boy,
wiggling and juggling his
big pot belly, what a funny jelly belly.

Tumble down to grin some more,
who's the earthquake maker
who's the walking walrus shaker
who's the smelly greasy fretter
the heaving panting layered sweater.

And we laugh those tons to come so near
with a curious twitch, our leery eyes meet
eyes with clouds and salty rains
eyes of booming lightening trains
eyes of storms with fire cores which
burn blue souls with Hades coals.

And I thought how dare he look to here
how dare that sloppy blubber baker
how dare that puffy whale scale breaker
how dare he look right here at me

Beep, beep, beep my pager sings
with white jacket, cross, and serpent pin
I head to doors of floors I reign
and with head held high and charts in hand
I knock and enter to see this man
and say, "Sir, what would you like to talk about?"

And he said
It's a foggy way
which I travel now
wish I had stayed
but I'm so hungry now
wish I'd bought more
shade and quiet place
with sounds of sticks and stones
with wounds which wear away.

And I said, "It sounds like you're lonely."
And he said, "It's how it's always been, doc."
And I said, 'How is your health?"
And he said, "The same as usual, doc."

"So, it says here in your chart that you were put on a weight reduction plan.

"Doc, you know I've had this discussion with you and your friends nine trillion times. I know my arteries are clogged and I can develop diabetes. There is nothing that works for me. I've tried it all."
"So, you're going to just give up. You're a quitter."

"Look doc, right now I'm feeling pretty sane; who knows when that's going to go away and I'll have a good old-fashioned breakdown for a little while or maybe for good. Let's be honest, what we're doing is just not working. I've stuck to my diet and nothing's changed. The medicine makes me sick, intestine bypass, gastric banding, jaw clamping, no thank you. My parents were both fat, though not as big as me and I swore I would never be like them."
"So, you're angry at your parents."

"No doc. I'm just saying I want you to treat my problem. Sure it's tough to go up three flights of steps, but I can deal with that. I want a better quality of life."

"Of course, and these surgeries in the right combination and with the right preparation will give it to you."
"Doc, why didn't *you* give it to me?"

"I don't know what you mean."

"Hey, doc, what would *your* quality of life be without your friends, your family, your girlfriend, your prestige, you know, your self-respect, doc?"

I said, "Self-respect is something that I get from within myself."

"Yeah, sure, doc. I'm pretty exhausted, I'll be heading home now."

And I said, "You know, it's all human nature anyway."

"So look who's the quitter now, doc."

Ajay Perumbeti

At the beginning of this creative piece, the young writer shares with us his numerous imaginings of the misery of the fat man as he was taunted and shunned throughout his life. He then moves on to reveal the moral insensitivity of the physician, and finally he leads us to witness the patient's ultimate resignation. This young writer compels us to imagine and feel with him the lifelong story of the fat man's suffering, and he ends the writing with palpable discomfort about not only the patient's impotence to resolve his problem, but his own.

Developing and Practicing Empathy

Although the basic skills of empathy are included in professional education, unfortunately they are infrequently practiced (28). Coulehan (28: 264–5) laments that ". . . our cultural suppression of empathy in medicine is anti-therapeutic . . . and has caused great dissatisfaction, anger, and unnecessarily bad outcomes." Exercises like those we have described earlier in this section – those that enable us to feel with the other, which work on us, and trigger our own emotions and sensitivities – are excellent techniques for developing and nurturing practitioners' empathic capacities.

This word "empathy" can be defined as the ability to understand and identify with another's emotional state (29). It derives from the German *Einfuhlung*, translated to mean feeling one's way into another person, an art form, music, etc. A family physician, William Zinn, explains how our modern term "empathy" encompasses a much broader context (30: 306):

> This process of feeling one's way into the experience of another is not limited to the emotional plane (i.e. the empathic individual does not, for example, merely experience along with the patient his sadness or joy). Instead he acts like more of a participant observer, resonating with the emotional and cognitive aspects of the experience and comparing them, both consciously and unconsciously, with his own relevant experience, memory, and fantasy.

From Zinn's words and those of others (30–33), clearly empathy has two dimensions – a cognitive dimension and an affective dimension. The cognitive dimension is the ability of the caregiver to take in and objectively understand the patient's experience and emotional state and then convey this understanding to her. The affective dimension is the ability to imaginatively feel what the patient feels. According to Kearny (34: 140), when ". . . we experience the suffering of other beings *as if* we were them . . . that provokes a reversal of our natural attitude to things and opens us to novel ways of seeing and being."

We asked the physician-poet John Stone about the meaning of empathy, and he brought to us the following two haiku poems (35: 10):

Empathy: You and I
Your veins connected
to my arteries, we breathe
and beat together.

John Stone

Empathy is a
house call from one human
spirit to another.

John Stone

In a few short phrases, Stone characterizes for us the close interconnections between two human beings resulting from the expression of compassion and empathy. In the clinical encounter, the medical professional's expression of empathy in a few words or short phrases has a profound therapeutic effect.

The patient feels that she has been heard and the practitioner understands her experience.*

Speaking about the importance of empathy, Frankel (37: 20) describes a communication process that is either helpful or faulty in this way:

> You start with a *potential empathic opportunity* – a hint of an emotion – and you [the caregiver] either terminate it, in which case the person is unlikely to bring it up again, or you move to an *empathic opportunity* by turning to wonder or engagement – simply being silent, being present, being curious, being interested. When the emotion comes, there's either an opportunity to terminate it or to pursue it. *If you pursue it, the patient, we think, feels understood.* (emphasis added)

Empathy significantly affects how patients accept and process difficult information. It is the key to establishing trust and rapport, and it supplies the framework for effective relationships. These assertions are reported in the results of a study by Wasserman and colleagues (38), and cited by Frankel (37), regarding the effect of emotional support (reassurance, encouragement, and empathy) during maternal care visits. The study (37: 18) concluded that "*Reassurances had no bearing on outcome whatsoever, nor did encouragement, but empathy was highly associated with visit satisfaction and reduction in maternal concern*" (emphasis added).

Empathy is not always expressed through verbal reflection of what the practitioner sees and feels in the patient. It can be conveyed through a simple enactment – attentive silence, a facial expression, a gesture, or a light touch on the arm. Patients judge an individual's empathic capability through the congruence of her verbal behaviors – that which she chooses to say – with her non-verbal behaviors such as her vocal tones and pitch, her facial expressions, and her posture. Intuitively patients know when empathy is present and when it is lacking.

In the medical encounter, the caregiver may not get the empathic response quite right. The patient, recognizing the attempt as genuine, may correct the caregiver and continue with her story. However, when the practitioner is not open to the information or correction given by the patient, or she ignores or misses emotional clues and fails to express empathy, the patient may close down. Halpern (33: iv), a psychiatrist and bioethicist, explains how this act of closing down can significantly impact medical work: "Missing important emotional cues from patients wastes time, leading to missed diagnoses, inadequate treatment adherence, and inadequate understanding of patient values in the face of tough medical decisions."

---

* The results of recent research (36) indicate a physiologic basis for a patient's positive response to a therapist's demonstration of empathy which provides some understanding for the human tendency to reflect or mirror each other's emotions.

Responding empathically requires mindful and imaginative listening and then reflecting back what you have heard. It is a teachable, learnable skill that requires committed, consistent practice. The following two exercises are effective methods of practice.

Empathic Response Practice: Dyads

Two people sit facing one another. One begins to tell an illness story or a story of some trauma in his life. The partner practices entering imaginatively into the teller's narrative and experiencing the feeling of the storyteller. The teller relates only a couple of lines and then pauses to allow his partner to respond empathically. There is no other questioning or commenting except for the empathic responses. This continues for about 5 minutes. Both people then discuss the responses and how to improve them. In this exercise, the workshop leader is circulating among the dyads and can be called to help when the need arises.

LLP

Empathic Response Practice: Group

Several people (six to eight) sit in a circle. One person is the leader and another person is the storyteller. The storyteller begins to tell her illness story, and at the leader's signal she stops. One person in the circle attempts to give an empathic response. The leader first asks the storyteller how the response felt. Discussion then centers on what kind of response it was. If it wasn't an empathic response, the focus switches to how to formulate a new response. Other people around the circle try their skill at responding empathically. The storyteller then resumes her story, and each time she stops, another person in the circle gives the first response, and the discussion continues until everyone has had an opportunity to respond and everyone has a clear understanding of what it means to respond empathically.

LLP

Until now in our discussion of empathy we have been concerned about the patient's experience, including her emotional status and the importance of compassionate and empathic care by health care professionals. We must also be concerned with the caregiver's emotional status in doing the work of medicine. Historically, trainees were warned routinely to remain detached from the emotional aspects of patient care in order to prevent loss of objectivity or becoming overwhelmed by the suffering of patients. Unfortunately, this admonition still occurs much too frequently. Burnout was and still is cited as a certain result. Detachment, the argument continues, would also prevent the heightening of patient emotion or the biasing of medical judgment which could result in impaired patient care. However, it is clear that the continual practice of repressing feeling and blunting one's affect results in demeanors that patients refer to as cold or uncaring (39). It is this very act of closing down that most often leads to burnout. Halpern (33: 10) posits that:

> . . . physicians' own emotions help them attune to and empathically understand patients' emotions. . . . The key issue is for physicians to become more reflective about their own emotional responses and learn to use those responses skillfully, rather than try to detach from them and be influenced by them anyway.

Medicine that is practiced with compassion, according to Coulehan (31: 232), demands emotional involvement, and requires skill in balancing what he describes as *tenderness* and *steadiness*. "The key issue then", Coulehan observes, "is being able to function in a *steady* or objective fashion, while also experiencing the emotional core of physician–patient interactions. I call this dual capability *emotional resilience.*"

Moral imagination and empathy are critical elements in medical work. Without them, we lack the ability to "feel our way into" our patient's being and to listen to her inner narrative. Without them, we work only on the surface, hearing and responding only to words, not to the whole meaningful story and the whole person who tells it.

Witnessing Personal Narratives

We conclude this section with a description of a complex exercise that combines training for three related skills – mindful listening, exercising moral imagination, and expressing empathy. The narrative writings that we share were crafted by three of us during an exercise in witnessing that was part of a narrative medicine workshop developed by Charon (40).* In this very rich task, each person is instructed to pair off with another, and each tells a story of a serious illness or traumatic or transformational event in her life. After hearing the story, the listener is asked to represent the story in writing and also to write how it felt to hear the other's story. Finally, the listener is asked to write reflectively about the story, and the storyteller is asked to write about how it felt to be listened to. We recount here our experiences with this exercise, as well as our own reflective writing that arose from this storytelling.

The story I (*JDE*) heard was told by a woman in her sixties about the birth of her child when she was a young woman. As far as she knew she was having a normal pregnancy. During childbirth and while she was still groggy from the sedation, her obstetrician told her, "We think your baby has Down's syndrome. But you can have another child." The storyteller related how hurt and angry she felt at the way he delivered the tragic news. Through the years, she and her husband loved their son deeply, but she was always aware that he was "not like others." As she tells the story, she wonders what prompts her crying:

---

* We are indebted to Dr Rita Charon and her team in the Program in Narrative Medicine at the College of Physicians and Surgeons of Columbia University for inventing this exercise.

An(other)

I should hear crying.
But through the anesthesia haze
I hear only screaming silence.

We suspect Down's
You can always have another.

How could you! How dare you!
Is this my error, to be erased by an(other)?
Why should he live? He's not like others.
But he must be –

Do what must be done, what can only be done
though he's not like others.

His father must be told.
His words wept anguish.
Engulfed in a hurricane of grief,
He returns to the classroom to teach others not like ours.

Now he's 10, still not like others.

Look at him! Your child is happy!

After all these years, these tears
Why?

He *is* happy.

JDE

My storyteller, through many tears, recounted to me (*LLP*) the death of her brother several years earlier in a skiing accident. At the time of his death, her mother could not deal with any part of it, withdrawing into the background, leaving my storyteller alone in her grief and solely responsible for the funeral arrangements:

Once Again

Mother called
She said, "David is no more."
What a strange thing to say.

Tragedy!
A skiing accident
Head trauma.
Only 19 years old
Too young to die
Yet he always seemed
To live on the edge.

Yes, I am 23 years old
But, oh no
Not ready to be responsible
For all this.
Where is Mother?

Once again I remember it all
Once again and once again and once again.

LLP

Charon's (41) purpose in sponsoring this workshop is to help medical professionals to understand important characteristics and outcomes that she describes as attention, representation, and affiliation. Our experience with this exercise reinforced our belief in the significant effect that compassionate presence and mindful listening (attention) have in our conversations with another person, and how sharing with the storyteller our reflective writing (representation) about their stories leads to a closer connection (affiliation) between the two participants. Each of our storytellers expressed feelings of gratitude at "being heard", and each was very pleased that we had captured their stories accurately and sensitively

READING AND INTERPRETING COMPLEX TEXTS

Jones (42) notes that early in the movement toward narrative medicine, when literary theorists such as herself, Trautman-Banks (43), Daniel (44), Hunter (45), Terry and Gogel (46), and Charon (47) heralded the benefits of reading literature to enhance clinical skills, they often referred metaphorically to the *patient as text* and the *physician as reader and interpreter.* Jones became concerned about the reductive nature of this idea, fearing that it could diminish the patient's story by giving authoritative voice to the physician. She cautioned (42: 192) ". . . to the extent that thinking of the patient as a text to be read and interpreted distracts physicians from remembering that patients are persons, not texts, the analogy contributes to the very reification and dehumanization of the patient that we in literature wanted to help counteract."

Today, many proponents of narrative medicine conceptualize the process as a dynamic *co-authoring* of illness stories – both are text, both are interpreters. The caregiver must enter the patient encounter possessing not only intellectual and technical expertise but also narrative skills which allow her to skillfully work with the patient to re-emplot a broken and inconsistent story into a coherent and insightful narrative.

How can health care professionals learn this act of co-construction and develop other skills critical to the practice of narrative medicine? Jones (48: 160) reasons that "Just as natural musical talent can be enhanced by the study and practice of music, narrative capacity can be enhanced by the study of literature and the interpretation of complex texts." We acknowledge that nearly any quality form of prose and poetry provides excellent and effective means for stimulating caregivers' skills in close reading and interpretation. However, in our short courses and seminars, we find that we capture participants' interest much faster and they tend to engage more fully if we use medically oriented materials – stories, essays, poems, and articles – in these programs. We broaden the mix of materials and include non-medically oriented works in our longitudinal programs.

Close reading and analysis of literary work requires focus and discipline. It places the reader inside the story where she becomes imaginatively engaged in the lifeworld of others, where she must analyze the interrelationships among the characters, deal with the ambiguity and vagary of the plot, and identify social and moral issues. Julia Connelly, a physician and strong proponent of the connections between literature and medicine, relates how literary characters enable practitioners to see patients from new perspectives (49: 151):

> As we listen to our patients, consider diagnostic possibilities, plan
> treatment strategies, and try to imagine the pain of another person,
> memories of others with similar symptoms come and go: memories
> that may offer reflections of literary characters as well as patients.
> Such memories add depth to our knowledge and possibilities to the
> directions of our interviews. We may more carefully search for hidden
> or unconscious feeling, for experiences that are difficult to share, and
> for common reactions that are considered *abnormal* by many.

In considerable detail, Charon (41) describes a *close reading* drill she has devised for training situations. She believes that the skills gained through the use of this technique stimulate medical professionals to examine patients' narrative texts more closely.* In practicing this drill, readers learn to identify five critical elements of a story:

1 the *frame* of the story – who is talking to whom about what, and what the teller wants in return for his narrative
2 the *form* of the story – the genre, structure and parts, and the characteristics of the narration and the narrator
3 the *time* of the story – how events occur and the folding and refolding of time
4 the *plot* – the action of the story, and the ordering of events into meaning
5 how the *desires* of the reader and the writer are satisfied – who has the need to tell and who has the need to know.

Charon (41) asserts that through the practice of close reading, the practitioner

---

* Readers can find a complete description of the drill in Charon's book *Narrative Medicine: Honoring the Stories of Illness* (41: 114–26).

will acquire skills which will effectively transfer to the patient interview. She will become more attuned to the patient's story and better able to understand the patient's perspective, and more effective in helping the patient to create meaning. Here are two techniques for enhancing the skill of close reading and interpretation.

Reading and Interpreting Literature

To demonstrate this technique, we chose our readers' theater adaptation of *The Death of Ivan Ilyich* to illustrate Charon's close reading process. The same commentary would apply to reading Tolstoy's original novella.

Form

Tolstoy's original work is in the form of a novella or short prose narrative, which takes place in the 1880s. Within this form are expositions on social and class life, the character of physicians, and the nature of medical care and caring relationships. The language is grave in nature and reflective of the time of its writing.

The narrator, one of the principal characters, guides the reader from the beginning of Ivan's professional and personal life through his increasingly successful professional life, his progressively dissatisfying married and family life, and finally to his death. We come to realize the complexity of the narrator as she changes during the course of the story. Early on, the narrator assumes a distanced and harshly critical posture toward Ivan. But over time she becomes more forgiving by getting closer to Ivan's lived experiences. In the last few acts of the play the narrator comes to empathize with Ivan's condition – his life trajectory. This affiliation allows the narrator to represent Ivan's most intimate thoughts and feelings to us.

Often one story will call to mind others. Charon (41) refers to this phenomenon as *intertextual conversations*. In reading *The Death of Ivan Ilyich*, we are reminded of the short story *Misery*, written by another well-known Russian author, Anton Chekhov. Just as no character in the story *Misery* wants to listen to the grief and loneliness of Iona Potapov, whose son dies, no one wants to listen to Ivan's grief and existential angst, and his feelings of desertion and isolation. Ivan's story reminds us also of the short story *Mercy* by Richard Selzer. In this story, the protagonist is dying of pancreatic cancer (Ivan was probably dying of the same disease), and we witness his suffering from uncontrollable pain. All of these stories raise important issues about the character of failed relationships between patients and their physicians.

Time

The retrospective of Ivan's life covers many years. However, the duration of time from his injury to his death appears to be measured in months. As in Tolstoy's original work, the scenes in the play encompass progressively shorter periods of time as Ivan approaches death. In the final scene, Ivan is just one hour from dying after three days of unremitting pain and screaming. In that hour he comes to an understanding of his life and he accepts death. The allegorical struggle between light and the "black sack of darkness" is brought to a close with Ivan's death.

Plot

Ivan Ilyich, a high-court judge in the city of St Petersburg, becomes seriously ill after injuring his side in a minor accident in his home. The author takes the reader from the time of a younger Ivan, "when life was good", to the dramatic and terrifying final stages of his dying. We witness the life choices that he makes to achieve success, and the effects of thoughtlessness and greed on him, his wife, his family, and friends. The physicians who minister to Ivan are deplorably inept, pompous, and uncaring. His family members, except for his son, are boorish, hypocritical, and cold. And his professional cohorts are self-absorbed. In the end Ivan receives graciousness, kindness and caring only from the house servant, Gerasim. He finally knows peace and healing when death overtakes him.

Frame and Desire

The author shows the reader how the lack of caring and compassion in a person's personal life seriously affects an otherwise successful and productive professional life. Tolstoy carefully traces Ivan's evolving frame of mind as the reader accompanies him through the fear, pain, and suffering that devastate his dying process, and the release that death finally offers. Although Ivan knows that he is dying, he cannot truly grasp it or accept it. When he finally realizes that the end is truly near, he begs to be released from his torment and fears the "falsity" of his life. In his final moments, when Vassili, his son, shows him love when no one else has done so, Ivan believes that he can still make his life "right." He knows it is time for him to die and to free them all – his family and his colleagues – from further trouble. Finally, the fear of death disappears and Ivan finds only peace and light and joy. In writing this story, is Tolstoy attempting to rid himself of his own fear of dying and convince himself that there is indeed a release in death? Does his new spiritual belief influence the story?

The skills developed through close reading enable a clinician to attend more closely to her patient and understand how the context, timing, and plot of the patient's story contribute importantly to her diagnosis, treatment, and life narrative. Under appropriate circumstances, this can lead to a closer and more wholesome affiliation.

Reading and Interpreting Poetry

Genuine poetry can communicate before it is understood.

T S Eliot (50)

The language beneath the language: this is poetry.

Andrea Pacione (51)

Often in a medical encounter the patient's story comes to the practitioner in bits and pieces. She listens and tries to find meaning in the patient's words and phrasings. As she works with her patient to fit the pieces together, the practitioner's reflective interior is constantly busy (this is *interior narration* as presented in Chapter 2). She formulates thoughts about the patient's story and determines how to respond. She compares perceptions and values, and decides to retain or change her own. She recalls the past actions and scenes of her own life that influenced her development. This activity of interior narration can also aptly be related to Eakin's process of lived biography described in Chapter 2. In this complex process of relating and negotiating, the practitioner makes initial judgments about the patient and her problem and speculates on a diagnosis.* Using another metaphor, the process of working with a patient's story becomes a dance – the patient and caregiver glide together, they dip, circle, and at times they trip over each other's feet as well as their own. One hopes to have a more meaningful story – even though it is incomplete – when the music fades. Terry and Gogel liken this interaction to the interpretation of poetry (46: 44):

> This tension between the meaning of the whole and the analysis of the parts is what is particularly well illustrated by the process of interpreting a poem. When looking at a poem, we may shift from concern regarding its ultimate meaning to a focus on such things as its tone, its voice, its shape and presentation on the page, or its energy level. We analyze these things as separate parts, although we infer them from the poem in its entirety.

Coulehan and Clary believe that reading, discussing, internalizing and writing poetry can help practitioners to become more reflective in a variety of ways (52: 384):

> For one, poetry teaches us the power of words, symbols, and metaphors to influence our patients. Having learned this, we are better able to modulate our interactions with them to promote healing. . . . Poetry also encourages the development of negative capability. A poem may have multiple and sometimes conflicting meanings. "Listening" to a poem often requires patience and respect. Finally, poetry fosters our ability to make the leap of empathy and, therefore, recognize our patients. Such recognition helps us to stand beside them in compassionate presence.

---

* Coulehan and Clary adopt Keats' term "negative capability" (52: 9) to describe the skill in considering and honoring uncertainties and doubts in one's mind at the same time.

In the light of the sentiments of all these authors, we look at three forms of poetry. First, let us consider the following poem, *Talking To The Family*, written by the physician–poet, John Stone (35: 6):

Talking To The Family

My white coat waits in the corner
like a father.
I will wear it to meet the sister
in her white shoes and organza dress
in the live of winter,

the milkless husband
holding the baby.

I will tell them.

They will put it together
and take it apart.
Their voices will buzz.
The cut ends of their nerves
will curl.

I will take off the coat,
drive home,
and replace the light bulb in the hall.

John Stone

In our initial reading of Stone's poem, we find that it does "communicate to us" and we do form an initial understanding of the overall meaning of the story. However, we are obliged to return for a second or third reading to "find the language beneath the language" and to closely examine how each part fits the whole and determine what it does. We want to learn who speaks to us and who holds the pain. As we grasp the fullness of all that Stone writes, we share with him the dread of donning the white coat hanging there in the corner, heavy now with the burden of delivering bad news to this family. We hear their voices and their tears, and then we feel with Stone the emptiness that follows.

Now, let us consider a brief prose poem written in one of our workshops by a mother, herself a medical practitioner:

Nearly eighteen years ago,
my son was being robustly examined
for brain surgery.
He had never spoken.
He and I had been away from home for three months
on this journey of finding help.

After one of the MRIs, the medical team met with us to review the
findings. As we spoke, I asked to see the images.
Kindly permitted, I gazed, and for a moment
found myself knowing my son as never before.
And I wept.
The physicians, one and all, watched and simply moved closer,
surrounding my son and me.

Anonymous

On first reading, the storyteller frames the story well for us. She carries us back
across many years to a critical moment in time, and we understand that she
wants us to know about the power of empathy. However, as with Stone's poem,
we return to probe the depths of her story further. We imagine how it was to
raise a child who doesn't speak, how it was to suffer alone the months of testing
and worry, and then how it was to "take in" the images through her eyes and
her heart. We hold her tears. And with her, we feel the empathy from the silent
circle of physicians surrounding her, and we sense the warmth and support she
felt at that moment.

We find haiku and other forms of Japanese poetry very effective in developing
practitioners' skills in imagination, focusing, and interpretation – skills that are
so important for clinicians. Marilyn Gustafson (53), a nurse educator, cites
the advantages of haiku – its ease and versatility which allow it to be used in
various situations and with different age groups, and the fact that it requires
no particular tools and can be combined with other media. Mary Anthony
(54:16), another nurse educator, proclaims that "Although writing haiku is not
an intense intellectual exercise, the inherent simplicity of this form of thinking
is what makes it so powerful." Haiku and other Japanese poetry forms – like a
painting or a photograph – are pure story, a moment of insight. Here are two
such poems:

my body
wasted by winter
if only I
like fields burned over
had hope for spring.

Lady Ise (55)

Empty-handed I entered the world
Barefoot I leave it.
My coming, my going –
Two simple happenings
That got entangled.

Kozan Ichikyo (56: 108)

In five short phrases Lady Ise reveals to us her yearning for more life to live as she faces her venerable age and inevitable death. Ichikyo's poem stimulates us to imagine life's narratives and relationships.

In both the reading and writing of haiku, we speculate on actual emotions that are not being expressed – a powerful key. We must search for meaning in the spaces between the written words, and also in the words that are not written. Asking medical professionals and trainees to read or to express their perceptions and feelings in haiku requires them to discard extraneous thoughts, their "one right diagnosis" sensibility, and to focus in on the exquisite meaning of the poem's core. In the medical interview, are these not the very skills that are vital for focusing closely on the meaning of what the patient is saying and all that is unspoken?

WRITING REFLECTIVELY AND TELLING COMPLEX CLINICAL STORIES

> I can still see you
> My first young patient to die
> Nothing I could do.
>
> *MD of 28 years*

Through habitual self-reflection we analyze our everyday lives, and consider our wisdom and our mistakes and the complexity of our relationships. Finding clarity about our beliefs and who we are empowers us to make the changes that we believe will help us to improve and to find existential meaning. The practice of honest self-reflection affects our relationships, our physical and mental health, our careers and lifestyle choices, our spiritual beliefs, how we judge and react to others' behaviors, and how we manage emotions.

Writing Reflectively

For clinicians, effective self-reflection and self-awareness are key factors in establishing effective relationships and providing competent and compassionate medical care. Practitioners benefit from continual self-questioning. In what ways might my ethnic and sociocultural background affect my work with my patients? How might my personal beliefs, values, and attitudes influence my patient care? What changes should I make to improve my interactions with others? Am I achieving my professional goals? What brings meaning to my work?

An effective exercise for stimulating caregivers' practice in self-reflection is to ask them to write in the voice of one of their patients how that person would describe them as a medical professional, and the quality of their relationship with them. The following is a piece written by a second-year resident.

My doctor, eh? Well, he seems pleasant enough, always smiling and what not. Sometimes I think he smiles a little too much, like maybe he's not all the way here but wants me to think he is. He certainly makes me feel like he's listening to me, but I get the sense he's in a hurry a lot, always shifting in his seat or writing something down in his chart. He's always telling me to call the office if I need anything, but I always end up talking to someone else. I guess that's part of him being busy. He lets me tell my stories, but sometimes I wish he wouldn't continue with the exam while I was talking. I'd rather see his eyes when I'm sharing these things. I know he wants the best for me, or at least it feels that way. It's hard to really believe that someone I've known over two or three 15-minute visits cares about me, even if it's supposed to be his job. Overall, I'm happy with my doctor. From what I hear from friends it could be a lot worse.

Israel Cajigas

This resident confronts his tendency to feign mindful attention and presence to his patient, and he sees himself exhibiting a harried demeanor, yet he believes that his patient will excuse his behavior because she knows that he cares about her, and another doctor could exhibit worse behaviors. Discussing his writing, he acknowledged the need to give his patients his full attention and to become more genuine in his interactions with others and himself.

Other narrative writing exercises that explore the patient's lived experience, the practitioner–patient relationship, or analyze personal experience and emotions also enhance clinical skills. When we ask participants to share their compositions orally, initially participants resist: "I don't have any talent. I can't write like Mary does." And invariably, although their creations are not always works of literary perfection, we find their compositions sensitive and heartfelt. In another document (57:32), we described the value of engaging students in writing reflectively as follows:

[Reflective] writing is one way of honoring the patient and preparing students to be both intimate and distanced with their patients. In listening and responding to the patient, the student develops an understanding of the patient's perspective. The student imaginatively puts herself in the patient's place and witnesses her perspective, ideas, emotions, anxieties, and suffering. This kind of deep understanding and intimacy requires the student not only to see the patient's reality but also to self-reflect and analyze her own reactions to "being in the patient's shoes." These characteristics allow the patient's illness narrative to be heard and brought to bear in their care. (insertion added)

Earlier in this chapter we described an exercise involving the use of portraits. We ask participants to imagine one of these people as their patient and to write a short paragraph describing their personal response to caring for the patient and what this indicates about their development as a caregiver. One participant chose to write about a gaunt, apparently very sick man:

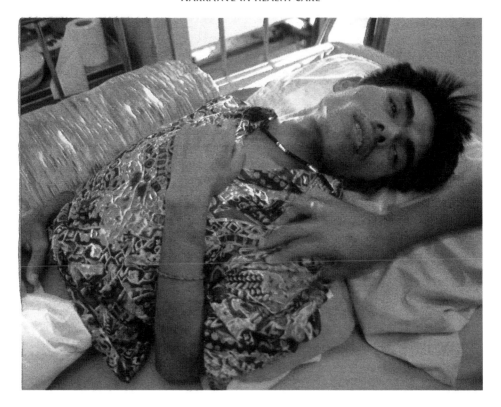

Immediately it is 1995 again. I am there again with my Dad as he lay dying of AIDS. As this patient talks, my Dad is all I can think about.

I find it almost impossible to listen to this patient's story.

Dad looked just like this – so thin, so weak, so tired of being sick.

I am overwhelmed. I cannot concentrate and focus on this patient. I wish I could, but I can't.

It is impossible.

Anonymous

In cogent descriptive language, this trainee painfully recalls her father's terrible illness and suffering. She laments how the memory occludes her own ability as a physician to deal with the suffering of this patient who is seeking her care. Her reflection has raised this caregiver's consciousness of how her own life experiences, when stirred up by her patient, can interfere with her attention to the patient's suffering. Awareness of this sort is critical to her formation as an empathic physician.

A second participant chose this photograph of a bright-looking, elderly woman.

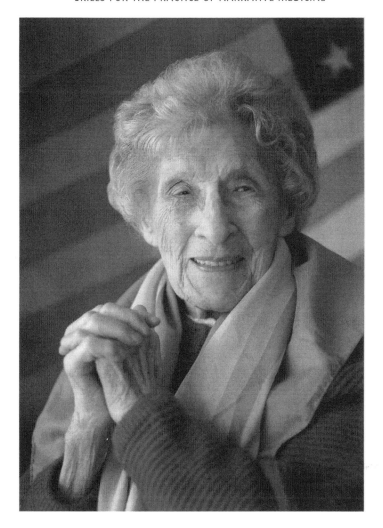

I feel privileged – I hear stories about days gone by that few get to hear. I am enriched by them.

I feel hopeless – that her memories will start to fade and I can do nothing to stop it, that her experience will be lost to the world.

I feel determined – to help her to maintain her dignity and independence in accordance with her wishes.

I feel humbled – that she could trust someone so young (compared to her) to care for her.

I feel mortal – I see her worn out body from head to toe and see myself in years to come.

Lynn Hamrich

In this piece a physician writes about her emotions while caring for this woman, but at the same time we hear her internal narration about her own identity as a physician. She reflects upon a set of complex feelings – the sense of privilege that medical work provides, her sense of obligation to be the keeper of her patient's stories, and her sense of determination, humility, and mortality so critical to her ability as a healer.

We also often invite patients who are willing to share their illness stories to join our class and allow trainees to conduct informal open group interviews with them. Following such a session, we ask participants to write in the voice of the patient. During one such interview, first-year medical students met Pete, a patient who had been diagnosed with amyotrophic lateral sclerosis (ALS). He was wheelchair-bound and possessed only minimal use of his right hand, with which he was able to manage the controls of his chair. He explained that in his first appointment following an extensive laboratory evaluation, the specialist whom he had met only once before walked into the consultation room and announced, "You'll be dead in six months." Pete related several experiences during his hospitalization and afterward that led him to renew his faith in God and, through the strength of his belief, his determination not to allow this disease to kill him. In a poem entitled *I'm Still Here*, one student highlights Pete's story poignantly. With passion, he captures the tension between the physician's detached view of Pete's disease and Pete's actual illness experience.

I'm Still Here

I'm still here
You don't seem to know it
Babbling on about diagnoses
And best treatment options with minimal cost
And when I will die.

I'm still here
You don't seem to care
I'm just another number
Another line in your appointment book
Who you think will die.

I'm still here
You don't seem to see me
Glancing at your watch
And minding your time
Scheduling when I will die.

I'm still here
You don't seem to hear me
Is your pager too loud
Or your mind too active
Deciding when I will die?

But I'm still here!
You may never know it
But there is more to life
Than your science, more to life than your ideas
And that is the part of me that will never die!

Robert Seese

When working with third-year medical students, we ask them to write about a patient they met in one of their clinical experiences. One student wrote imaginatively in the voice of a 24-year-old patient who came to the Emergency Room after a fainting episode. She had fainted 15 to 20 times before and had never seen a doctor about this. The patient's medical history included bipolar disorder and the use of crack cocaine. She had been hospitalized in the psychiatry unit four times. She was the single parent of two young children, and her story involved sexual abuse. The student "finds her way into" the patient's illness narrative, her physical and spiritual suffering, her wonder at being a parent, and the torment of her affliction.

I am feeling alone and tired, what a long day. All these people wanting so much from me and I'm not sure I can come through. I have so much to do and I feel like it will never get done. How did I get here and how will I survive? How did my life end up like this? It seems like everyone else has it so easy. One day I'm in high school having fun with no responsibilities, and now I'm in charge of three people and barely surviving. I know my life is good – I am alive and my children are here with me, but still I am overloaded. I need to escape, I need something to help me, just to help me relax. No, Julie, you have to stop thinking about this, you must concentrate on your new life, not the old one. You are doing a good job, hang in there.

Wow, she is beautiful and she's mine. What a great picture of us. What an honor really to have her love me, that should be enough. These pictures of us are so cute and she looks like me, her mommy. I wonder what her life will be like? Can I raise her? Will I be good enough and keep her out of trouble? Oh God, here comes the feeling. It's getting closer and closer. I can't push it away. Oh God, I can't breathe. Calm down, you will be fine. No, I won't, I can't handle this. Too much, way too much . . . I can't breathe, can't feel my hands. . . . Oh, God.

Mommy! Mommy! Wake up!

Hey, Julie, wake up, come back to us.

Emily Gale

The following poem, *The Mountain*, was written by a first-year medical student who had interviewed a woman suffering from multiple sclerosis (MS). He told the class how he himself felt the incredible weight of her disease as she described her life. She was no longer a woman *with* MS, she *was* MS. He captures the woman's terrible plight and her dis-ease in his poem, and we feel the weight that he felt. Notice how the student positions his phrases to emphasize the meaning.

The Mountain

It's like you're   all alone
        Flying a plane
               that slams into the side of a mountain
A mountain.

A mountain called MS sprang up outta nowhere
      swallowed the horizon and BAM!
      reduced my life to smoke and tears and
      screams and broken glass.

I used to be a teacher ya know
elementary school
    before the crash
    before the mountain
        took everything and
        left me like this.

Gone is the classroom, gone are the kids, gone
Are all the apples
        just never enough
        apples to keep the
        doctors away.

I know what you're thinking
I don't even look sick, right?
Why don't You try going to sleep at night
        trembling from fear
        afraid that tomorrow
        you might wake trembling
        from something else.

I didn't ask for this, OK?
        I don't ask "why me?"
But I didn't ask for this
        I ... I ... never ask "why me?"

I want to go on living. I want to have fun. I want
the silver lining. I really do.
But this demon that slipped inside me
shoots across my nerves
A fork of lighting

innocently dancing electric wires
stabbing at balance
dispersing control
leaving everything a mess.
This demon that's now a mountain
too big not to overwhelm
erased the sun
became my field of vision
lost in its frigid shadow
all that I can see.

Phoenix Ho

In discussing these writings, we address many of the elements of Charon's close reading drill. We ask each author to talk about what they wrote and why they chose to portray the material in the particular way that they did.

Listening to and Telling Stories in a Group

Just as important as writing reflectively is the act of telling stories to one another or in a community setting. Greenhalgh reflects on this as she writes (2: 40):

> Intra-group discussion about what a particular story *means* fuels the learning cycle, especially if skilled facilitation prompts the group to seek knowledge from external sources (experts, books, or databases) at the critical point in the cycle.

As we mentioned, participants in our workshops often express some initial reluctance about sharing their creation. However, this generally disappears after the first person has contributed. Understandably, sharing stories in a group prompts comments and questions about appropriate medical treatment and outcome, but it also generates valuable discussion about how the clinician felt about the particularities of caring for this patient at this time in this way. Listening to a complex clinical story is vastly different from hearing a concisely stylized case presentation stripped of emotional or ethical complexity. Some stories draw respectful contemplative silence, while others prompt heartfelt or muted emotions – anger, mirth, or sadness. Jones points out that raising the storyteller's awareness about her "telling" style can influence how one listens. She explains how sharing stories can improve narrative competence (48: 161):

> The writing and oral telling of complex clinical and ethical texts are routinely required of clinicians and ethicists as they carry out their work. Whether they realize it or not, in writing or presenting cases, they make stylistic choices that influence the way their own stories will be read and interpreted. Becoming aware of such stylistic choices and the effects these choices have on readers' or listeners' comprehension

and interpretation – even on patients' compliance – is an important
step in developing narrative competence.

As Jones states above, stories carry the perceptions of the storyteller, and
storytellers have different perceptions of the same character or event. Telling
stories and comparing stories in a group setting helps to train caregivers to listen
closely. Equally important, it enables participants to explore different feelings and
interpretations, different values, different approaches and procedures, and new
ways of thinking. Sharing and comparing reactions broadens participants' views
of patients and illnesses and enhances their own professional development.

Reflective writing that is derived from group interviews with one patient is
compelling and revealing. All of the students in the group hear the same story,
yet their reflective writings often present widely varied views on the patient's
life experience. Each story is told from a particular perspective, assumes certain
interests, and envisions certain outcomes (5). It is instructive for students to
hear these varied interpretations and discern how each student brings her own
values, biases, and personhood to these writings.

In one session with a patient, students met Alan, an elderly man who was
suffering heart failure due to severe cardiomyopathy. Alan described his career
as an aviation engineer, his illness, and his concern for his wife of many years,
and he spoke of his children, some of whom were now estranged. The following
story pieces are drawn from narratives written by two different students from
this same patient interview.

> . . . your life is not predictable. . . . Looking at you, I never would have known that
> you go out in a canoe on the weekends just to look at the beauty of nature. I never
> would have known that you had a special spiritual encounter when you were lying
> on your back in pain. It really showed me once again how no one is a statistic. At the
> same time, you were very ordinary. . . . If I walked into a grocery store, I never would
> have noticed you standing behind me with your cart full of fresh vegetables and
> that special steak for Friday night. I don't think of you as being too much different
> from my own grandfather.

> . . . I was touched to be a medical student on that night. It made my life's work
> seem that much more worthwhile because an elder of the community took the time
> to give his special wisdom to me. It means a lot to me that I'm going to become
> someone very seriously able to help others in such a deep way. But I won't forget
> your advice, Alan. I'll remember not to force my views onto others. I'll be open when
> others want to know why I do things the way I do. And every time they do want to
> know, I'll think of you, Alan.

> *Justin Kunes*

You were once a scientist, you told me so. You helped build planes, missiles, vehicles

that kept me safe while I was too young to know

that the world is not always a perfect place.

Now I am becoming a scientist, to keep others safe.

However, my art cannot save you now – five years or less.

What is the justice in that?

Michael Cowher

The first student contemplates multiple facets of the interview – the ordinariness of this man who seems to live quite serenely with a condition that can kill him at any moment, his own identity as a physician-in-training, and the powerful lessons he has been taught by his "knowing" this patient. In the second composition, the student laments the impotence of his profession's "science" in the face of the patient's dire condition. Hearing such different stories based on the same interview allows participants to understand that representation of a life at any single point in time is only one perspective, partially correct and partially understood.

Each of the stories presented above demonstrates that the writers have been effectively challenged, through reflection, to share in the lived experience of another, and have connected that experience with their own emotions and reactions. Many students and health care professionals in our courses and workshops possess considerable talent for writing creatively. Others may be less gifted, yet their writing demonstrates that they have indeed imagined and entered into the lifeworld of the other. They reveal a deepened sensitivity to their patient's suffering, and capture the essence of the patient's interior narrative. When we discuss how trainees feel about such exercises, the most common response is "I feel much closer to the patient." And when students share their writings with the patients, these people without exception feel honored, empowered, and also emotionally closer to the student. Certainly this kind of testimony gives credence to the notion that reflective writing, despite its difficulty for some, is of worth for both practitioners and patients, and for their relationships.

REASONING WITH STORIES

The use of narrative – to incite people to think critically, to teach social attitudes, to transmit culture and history, or to strengthen particular moral beliefs – has been taking place since the time of primitive humankind, and continues in all cultures (34, 58–60). As very young children we learn how to reason through stories told by our parents and grandparents, through nursery rhymes, through fairy tales, and through our first books. Through stories we learn right from wrong, how to make correct decisions, and how to live congenially with others.

At the beginning of Chapter 1, we encountered a powerful clinical story depicting an experience that dramatically affected both the physician and his patient. We invite you to consider the story of the patient parallel to the story of the physician, to envision the outcome that each participant faced, and to discern the interpretive influences that are at play. The story prompts still further questions. How are the professionalization and/or socialization of the impressionable young medical students and the residents affected? What is the transformative twist in the story and who was transformed? What self-knowledge might the participants derive from the story? Exploring this story and the questions that we pose is an example of an exercise in narrative reasoning. Frank (61: 23) refers to this process as ". . . thinking *with* stories as opposed to the more conventional academic and scientific approach of thinking *about* stories." It is an activity that Morris describes (60: 196) as one ". . . in which we as thinkers do not so much work on narrative as take a radical step back, almost a return to childhood experience of allowing narrative to work on us."

Stories that trigger our emotions prompt us to analyze what we think and feel about the issues disclosed in the story, and may influence the way we make decisions and how we act at some other time. When the physician in our opening story finally hears how his patient's life has been disrupted and he allows his emotions to surface, he is moved to view the situation differently, and we observe a critical shift in his moral stance. With regard to the role that emotions play in our cognition, Morris quotes philosopher Martha Nussbaum (60: 209): "We discover what we think . . . partly by noticing how we feel; our investigation of our emotional geography is a major part of our search for self-knowledge." Morris summarizes (60: 209): "Self-knowledge is indispensable to a moral life, and thus ethical conduct is impossible or fatally impaired without an investigation of feeling."

Although there is increasing emphasis today on the teaching of values and attitudes in our professional schools, the teaching of knowledge and skills still remains the primary focus. Hence when graduates enter clinical arenas and are immediately confronted with the ubiquitous moral and ethical dilemmas presented there, they are too often bereft of effective skills for dealing with them. Certainly stories are an integral part of clinical work, but more often they are stories of disease or scientific and technical application, rather than stories that compel reasoning about beliefs, values, and morals. In professional education in particular, narrative reasoning exercises are one way to refocus attention on the critical dimensions of stories involving both caregivers and their patients. As Hensel and Rasco assert (62: 500):

> [The] object is not to teach students rules to live by, but to help
> them make rules that are at once their own and in keeping with the

profession's tradition . . . storytelling creates the kind of atmosphere that encourages continuous improvement and provides a means of helping students interpret their experiences based on their individual personalities and personal beliefs.

By sharing his story in Chapter 1, *JZ* provides a forum in which young physicians and students can examine and temper their own feelings of incompetence or guilt about particular patient experiences they have encountered. In support of this idea, Hensel and Rasco write (62: 503):

> Using stories and storytelling helps students deal with immediate situations, such as patient encounters that are currently troubling them. By being immediate, practical, and specific, appropriate stories have the best chance of influencing the values and beliefs of those who hear them.

When working with third-year medical students during their clinical rotations, we invite them to participate in their patients' narratives, imagining their lived experiences. We ask them to write in the patient's voice, the patient's interior dialogue, to express what the patient is experiencing as a result of illness and medical care. The students then share and discuss their writing. An exercise of this nature provides an opportunity for all participants to share experiences and consider their own feelings, values, and beliefs about each story that they tell and hear.

One student introduced her patient as follows. The patient is a 78-year-old retired pediatrician with prostate cancer and benzodiazepine abuse. He was driven to his doctor's office by his son after being found that morning lying on the floor with a gash over his eyebrow. His son reported increasing forgetfulness and frequent falls over the past two years. The patient was unable to recall the events that led up to his fall, so the history was obtained from the son. The student writes imaginatively in the patient's voice:

What brings you into the office today, Dr Roe?, the medical student asked me.

I have good blood pressure. I always have good blood pressure. It's never been high, I told her proudly.

He forgets a lot of things nowadays, his son explained somewhat sadly.

I do. Details. Details. Moments of clarity. Flashes from the past. I used to teach these medical students. I used to dazzle them. I taught them how to care for small bundles of love who would grow to be adults. We were all part of a team.

How are you today, Miss? The medical student looked at me blankly for a second and then muttered something along the lines of an apology for her hesitancy. The residents and medical students, we all had bad days. But most of us didn't show it.

Does she know that I understand, doctor to doctor, or does she think that I am just an old man being polite? Am I still part of the team?

What made you decide you wanted to become a doctor? my interviewer had asked. When I was little, I wanted to be an artist. In grade school, I realized the importance and the impact my teachers had upon me. Good or bad. I wanted to be one of the good ones. When I fell in love with Sara, I knew I wanted to be a father. When I became a father, I realized I wanted to become a protector, a healer. I cried the day Blake was born. Our own little bundle of love. It's been so long since we've played baseball. And now, how he looks after both of us. I wish things could be different. He has children of his own to watch grow up. I miss getting dressed up and taking Sara out to nice restaurants. I miss dancing. Oh, how she could make me feel so alive. I miss her.

This terrible disease. It is taking away all my memories. They say I will forget who my wife and son are. I will become a body without memories. Part of a person. Who will remember my memories if I cannot? Who will remember the feeling I had on my wedding day or the romantic dinners Sara cooked for me after a hard day at work? Who will remember those father-son fishing trips? Or the excitement I felt when I graduated from medical school? But I've had a full life. I suppose in my experiences I have always thought the ending of a life for a young child to be more tragic than that of an old man. My work lives in those I have healed, those who will continue to teach the way I taught them. My emotions live in those I loved.

I'll be right back, Dr Roe. I'm going to hunt down an otoscope.
Thank you, I whispered quietly.

Karen Ho

When this story was shared in the group, the students commented on the powerful question invoked by the physician–patient: "Am I still part of the team?" They noted the strangeness of having a physician as a patient, and how it strips away his identity and turns him into a much more vulnerable and helpless person whose "value" in the world may be hidden to his caregivers. His aging and his illness have disconnected him from his medical teaching team which he used to "dazzle", and have disconnected him from the human team as well. His fading memories begin to extinguish his own son and wife from his personhood, and he is diminished to become just a "body", only "part of a person." The students became engaged in discussion of ways that they could attempt to reconnect this patient to the people and things that gave his life meaning. The discussion created a greater consciousness of the lived experience of illness from the patient's perspective. We believe that the telling and hearing of stories such as these is critical to the professional development of young physicians, nurses, and other practitioners. How they process these experiences and what they see their colleagues and their teachers do in these stories shape their sense of how they want to be in their caring for others.

ENGAGING IN NARRATIVE ETHICS

What is narrative ethics? One answer to this question is that, like virtue-based ethics, it is a remedy for the perceived limitations of principle-based ethics. Narrative approaches to medical ethics* are based on two related beliefs. One is that moral principles are not universal and law-like when applied to human systems, but contingent in the light of particular contexts. The other is that the particulars of human situations follow a narrative form and have a narrative structure in order to have moral meaning. Another response to the question is what the ethicist Tom Murray has argued (63). It is possible to think about narrative as moral education, methodology, discourse, and justification. In this chapter, we focus on narrative ethics as a methodology for informing moral judgments through a process that is based on a connection among reasoning with stories and exercising moral imagination and empathy. The basis for this complex form of narrative ethics is found in the ideas of Aristotle and Kant. Although the detailed arguments for these connections are beyond the scope of this chapter, we encourage the interested reader to examine Richard Kearney's work *Poetics of Imaging: Modern to Post-Modern* (64), particularly the epilogue to his book. With regard to narrative ethics, the focus in this chapter is on understanding moral dilemmas. We use the following story as an introduction to thinking about narrative ethics.

I was the Pastoral Care Volunteer assigned to the ICU. Because most patients in this unit were intubated and often comatose, I generally ended up attending patients whose family members were at the bedside. One of the beds held an elderly comatose man attached to numerous tubes and lines and blinking machines. Late one afternoon, I found three women surrounding his bed – an elderly wife/mother in a wheelchair pulled close to the bed, one daughter standing beside her, and a second daughter on the opposite side of the bed. Clearly, the two younger women were arguing. One was crying, and the other was looking angry and determined. *It's time to let him go*, said the crying sister. *No, that is not what he would want*, claimed the other. Their mother, exhausted, forlorn, with tears sliding down her wrinkled cheeks, looked from one to the other and then laid her head down on the side of the bed next to her husband. Obviously they were arguing about life support. *But you heard his doctors – they don't think he will come out of this*, said one sister. *No! I tell you! He would want to continue. He would not quit! All my life, he always insisted, you don't give up, you keep working and you will get where you want to go. That's how he got me through college. He would never give up!*, said the other.

LLP

---

* There are several members in the narrative ethics family, such as feminist ethics, care-based ethics, and relational ethics. Narrative is fundamental to all of these ethical viewpoints. A cornerstone of all viewpoints is the value placed on the particulars of the patient's story. What separates particular viewpoints in this family is the addition of other social and/or political values to a narrative core.

In this scenario, the emotions of the two sisters run high while the wife/mother finds herself stranded and impotent. How can this dilemma be resolved? What is the "right" thing to do? Will someone bear resentment, perhaps forever? What role will the medical professionals assume?

Some practitioners – those who favor principle-based ethics – prefer to use analytical reasoning to make judgments based on principles which they have stored from previously learned and universally accepted theories and precepts, and disallow their emotions to "muddy" the process. According to them, all cases should be decided objectively and with analytic conformity. In contrast, Greenhalgh argues (2: 92), ". . . in narrative ethics (sometimes known as existential or virtue ethics), the emotional reaction to the case – to the characters, actions, and events in the story – is *part of the process* of reaching an ethical decision." Whereas *principlists* tend to operate in a linear, somewhat autocratic format (a situation which may prevent the patient or family from correcting misinformation or entering the decision process), narrative ethics places decision making in the context of the patient's life story. Shapiro and Ross highlight this point (65: 99): "A narrative approach does not involve physician persuasion or coercion. Rather, it encourages the patient to find his/her own voice and to make choices about how he/she wants to live."

As practitioners of narrative medicine, our work requires us to develop the kind of relationships with our patients that enable us to formulate mutually acceptable and ethically sound decisions. Brody considers that we can only accomplish this through the *joint construction of narrative*. He states (66: 85): "One important element of the joint construction of narrative is that the patient is fully involved throughout the whole process. The physician does not hand the new narrative . . . to the patient in the way that the traditional physician hands out a prescription at the end of a visit." Instead, he engages in what Brody (66) and Gadow (67) term a *relational ethic*. Interestingly, Launer (5) likens the narrative construction process to a circular *three-dimensional dance* as opposed to a typical linear model that has a specific diagnosis and treatment plan. In Launer's construct, the patient and practitioner co-author stories that are not static. They have no beginnings or endings, they contain many feedback loops, and potentially they can evolve into something new.

How do we go about working toward an ethical solution for the dilemma that we encountered in the ICU? Greenhalgh (2: 42) urges us to ". . . consider the ethical problem as a *story*. Who are the actors? What has happened so far? What will be the consequences of different courses of action? How do we *feel* about those consequences?" There are four actors in the ICU story – the patient, who now lies comatose and on life support, the elderly wife/mother, and her two daughters, who have sidelined and silenced her as they vehemently disagree over whether to continue or discontinue life support for their father. Continuation of life support possibly leads to a long-term vegetative state and a slow deterioration for the patient, accompanied by high financial and emotional costs for the family. The wife/mother is elderly. How will this affect her physical and emotional health? Termination of life support may shorten the immediate suffering of all involved, but will there be far-reaching spiritual suffering for one or more of the actors? Perhaps the most reasonable way to reach a decision in this dilemma is for all three women to come together with a practitioner who will create a neutral yet compassionate environment where they can safely explore their values, the meaning of their stories, and the sources of their feelings. In this forum they need to discuss the consequences of the two options, share their feelings about the consequences and, weighing all factors one against the other, decide on an action that each can accommodate in their lives.

In a similar vein, Smith (68), a professor of human values, proposes a narrative approach in which the health care team, family members, and patients come together to share stories about the particular situation, interpret together the meaning of the stories, and try to arrive at a decision that is acceptable to all. He offers the following listing of narrative prompts which caregivers can use to approach ethical problems (68: 5):

1   Understand your own story. How do you see the characters and events? What future does your story imply? What values does it reveal? What are virtues in the characters?
2   Encourage others involved to tell you their stories. Understand patients', family members' and other caregivers' perceptions and values by listening to their stories. Interpret their stories as you did your own.
3   Encourage the elaboration of key events and characters to make the stories more complete and revealing.
4   Clarify facts in the stories where they are inaccurate or unclear.
5   Examine analogies for the appropriateness of the comparison. Offer alternative analogies where appropriate.
6   Encourage the elaboration of future episodes implied by the stories told. Note where different and similar futures are implied by different stories.
7   Encourage those involved to share stories and to pool their stories toward accuracy, completeness, coherence, unity, and a good fit with experience.
8   Offer alternative future episodes where appropriate.
9   Develop a story which integrates the values of those involved, implies an acceptable future, and guides actions.

Clearly an important element of narrative competence is the ability to discover all that stories can tell us. As we have suggested, writing stories is an interpretive event. So, too, is the telling of stories. As others have noted (2, 48, 58, 68), we generally learn as much about the storyteller as we do about the story events. Stories tell us about the implicit values and beliefs of the storyteller and how they serve as foundations and justifications for actions. This understanding allows clinicians to search for and comprehend how and where ethical and moral issues are embedded in patients' stories.

Earlier in this chapter we described how movies and videos can provide stories to challenge caregivers' moral imagination. They are equally valuable as sources of stories to stimulate ethical thinking in narrative contexts. To demonstrate the use of film for this purpose, we return once again to the video, *A Choice for K'aila*. We noted that this film documents the dilemma facing a Canadian family in accepting or refusing a liver transplant for their baby boy. After viewing the video and discussing the attitudes of the characters and the ethical dimensions of the story, we ask participants to write reflectively in the voice of one of the characters. Interestingly, two young trainees wrote from the perspective of the doctor. The first is an expression of lament for the unyielding position that the doctor assumed by urging the transplantation – a position which inevitably caused terrible emotional pain for K'aila's parents, and which now gives rise to serious emotional pain in himself. The second piece describes the moral conflict that the doctor might feel in having to make this medical decision and in considering the parents' concerns.

I can't seem to find the words
to express the loss I feel.
I know I'd die a thousand deaths
for the chance for you to heal.

I regret the nights you will not spend
staring at the stars
or traveling with your family
or buying your first car.

Your parents seem to understand
and handle it far better than I.
Despite my best efforts
I was forced to watch you die.

I'm sorry for the pain I caused.
I was not strong enough to let go.
In the end you left too soon,
and forever that I will know.

Max Safder

How can I allow this to happen? It is my duty to this infant to give him whatever chance I can. I understand where his family is coming from and the beliefs they hold. But how can I just remain inactive? What if this is not what he would have wanted? Someone else has to weigh in on this. But I wonder if it is as much for my own benefit as it is for his. Never playing in the yard, never climbing a tree, never seeing a sunset, never falling in love – how can he be deprived of these things? I know nothing in medicine is certain, but shouldn't I at least give this kid a chance? These parents are either the most callous monsters on the planet or more loving than I could imagine. Sometimes I am so torn that I can't be sure what I'm seeing in them.

Israel Cajigas

Clearly, these residents comprehend the significance of the intense situations that are presented in films such as *A Choice for K'aila,* and are able to organize and find meaning in the tragic events in the lives of the characters that they portray. Although it is an empirical question, it does seem reasonable to speculate that these narrative skills should transfer to the care of patients and self. It is our hope that later in their careers these caregivers will be better equipped to counsel a patient or a younger colleague when confronted with a similar ethical situation.

A TRANSFORMATION

We close this chapter by taking one last look at our initial storyteller from Chapter 1. With considerable distress, he came to an important realization about his patient's suffering and his own shortcomings as a caregiver. Let us imagine that he has worked with us on the six narrative skills. How does he appear to us now? Has he changed?

We see him becoming a more skilled architect of the therapeutic relationship. He has learned how to work more effectively with his patient to construct a whole new story, not missing the information about the importance and love of piano playing in the patient's life. He avoids making an unethical decision about treatment because together he and the patient decide on a procedure that avoids disabling surgery. Rather than denigrating the patient's whining, he expresses empathy and commends the strength and courage that his patient demonstrates in this troubling situation. He remains present to the patient's suffering, knowing that his emotional engagement will likely have a therapeutic effect on them both. The challenges faced by this physician are still difficult and at times overwhelming, but with a quieter mind and spirit he finds new ways of thinking and imagining, and he increasingly trusts his creative abilities. The patient recognizes and appreciates that a new dimension of relationship – an affiliation – is beginning to develop between them. He feels that the physician pays more attention to what he says and gives him more treatment options to consider. In turn, the physician feels greater satisfaction with himself, his capabilities, and his career. In short, a transformation is taking place.

FURTHER ACTIVITIES

Readers who are interested in learning more about the various techniques discussed in this chapter are encouraged to consult the following:

- Savitt TL. *Medical Readers' Theater: a guide and scripts.* Iowa City, IA: University of Iowa Press; 2002.
- Dobie S. Reflections on a well-traveled path: self-awareness, mindful practice, and relationship-centered care as foundations for medical education. *Acad Med.* 2007; **82:** 422–7.
- McDrury J, Alterio M. *Learning Through Storytelling in Higher Education: using reflection and experience to improve learning.* London: Kogan Page; 2002.
- Greenhalgh T, Collard A. *Narrative-Based Healthcare: sharing stories – a multiprofessional workbook.* London: BMJ Books; 2003.
- Higginson WJ. *The Haiku Handbook: how to write, share, and teach Haiku.* New York: Kodansha International; 1985.
- Reichhold J. *Writing and Enjoying Haiku: a hands-on guide.* New York: Kodansha International; 2002.
- Kabat-Zinn J. *Coming to Our Senses: healing ourselves and the world through mindfulness.* New York: Hyperion; 2005.
- Kabat-Zinn J. *Full Catastrophe Living: using the wisdom of your body to face stress, pain, and illness.* New York: Dell Publishing; 1990.
- Kornfield J. *Meditation for Beginners.* Boulder, CO: Sounds True; 2004.
- Brady M. *The Wisdom of Listening.* Boston, MA: Wisdom Publications; 2003.

REFERENCES

1 Charon R. Literary concepts for medical readers: frame, time, plot, desire. In: Hawkins AH, Chandler MM, editors. *Teaching Approaches to Literature and Medicine.* New York: MLA Publications; 2000. pp. 29–41.
2 Greenhalgh T. *What Seems to be the Trouble? Stories in illness and healthcare.* Oxford: Radcliffe Publishing; 2006.
3 Greenhalgh T, Hurwitz B. Why study narrative? In: Greenhalgh T, Hurwitz B, editors. *Narrative-Based Medicine.* London: BMJ Books; 1998.
4 Charon R. *Narrative Medicine;* http://litsite.alaska.edu/healing/medicine.html
5 Launer, J. *Narrative-Based Primary Care.* Oxford: Radcliffe Medical Press; 2002.
6 Connelly J. Being in the present moment: developing the capacity for mindfulness in medicine. *Acad Med.* 1994; **74:** 410–14.
7 Dobie S. Reflections on a well-traveled path: self-awareness, mindful practice, and relationship-centered care as foundations for medical education. *Acad Med.* 2007; **82:** 422–7.
8 Epstein RM. Mindful practice. *JAMA.* 1999: **282:** 833–9.
9 Sakalys JA. Restoring the patient's voice: the therapeutics of illness narratives. *J Holist Nurs.* 2003; **21:** 228–41.
10 Moyne B, Barks C. *Unseen Rain: quatrains of Rumi.* Boston, MA: Shambala; 2001.
11 Rinpoche CN, Shlim DR. *Medicine and Compassion.* Boston, MA: Wisdom Publications; 2006.
12 Ram Dass, Gorman P. The listening mind. In: Brady M, editor. *Wisdom of Listening.* Somerville, MA: Wisdom Publications; 2003.

13 Levinson W. Mining for gold. *J Gen Intern Med.* 1993; **8:** 172.

14 Shafir RZ. *The Zen of Listening.* 2nd ed. Wheaton, IL: The Theosophical Publishing House; 2003.

15 Kabat-Zinn J. *Full Catastrophe Living: using the wisdom of your body and mind to face stress, pain, and illness.* New York: Dell Publishing; 1990.

16 Kabat-Zinn J, Massion AO, Kresteller J *et al.* Effectiveness of meditation-based stress reduction program on the treatment of anxiety disorders. *Am J Psychiatry.* 1992; **149:** 936–43.

17 Speca M, Carlson LE, Gooday E *et al.* A randomized wait-list controlled clinical trial: the effect of a mindfulness meditation-based stress reduction program on mood and symptoms of stress in cancer outpatients. *Psychosom Med.* 2000; **62:** 613–22.

18 Schneider RH, Staggers F, Alexander CN *et al.* A randomized controlled trial of stress reduction for hypertensive older African Americans. *Hypertension.* 1996; **28:** 228–37.

19 Costello-Richmond A, Schneider RH, Alexander CN *et al.* Effects of stress reduction on carotid atherosclerosis in hypertensive African Americans. *Stroke.* 2000; **31:** 568–73.

20 Kabat-Zinn J, Litworth L, Buaney R *et al.* Four-year follow-up of a meditation-based program for the self-regulation of chronic pain and treatment outcomes and compliance. *J Pain.* 1986; **2:** 159–73.

21 Reibel DK, Greeson JM, Gainard GC *et al.* Mindfulness-based stress reduction and health-related quality of life in a heterogeneous patient population. *Gen Hosp Psychiatry.* 2001; **23:** 183–92.

22 Johnson M. *Moral Imagination.* Chicago, IL: University of Chicago Press; 1993.

23 Kleinman A. *The Illness Narratives.* New York: Basic Books; 1988.

24 Weine SM. The witnessing imagination: social trauma, creative artists, and witnessing professionals. *Lit Med.* 1996; **15:** 167–82.

25 Sarbin TR. The role of imagination in narrative construction. In: Davide C, Lightfoot C. editors. *Narrative Analysis.* Thousand Oaks, CA: Sage; 2004.

26 Clelow C. Imaginative writing. *Med Educ.* 2001; **35:** 1152–4.

27 Canadian Broadcasting System. *A Choice for K'aila.* Man Alive Series; 1992.

28 Coulehan J. Empathy and narrativity: a commentary on "The origins of healing: an evolutionary perspective of the healing process". *Fam Syst Health.* 2005; **23:** 261–5.

29 Hirsch EM. The role of empathy in medicine: a medical student's perspective. *Med Educ Virtual Mentor.* 2007; **9:** 423–7.

30 Zinn W. The empathic physician. *Arch Intern Med.* 1993; **153:** 306–12.

31 Coulehan J. Tenderness and steadiness: emotions in medical practice. *Lit Med.* 1995; **14:** 222–36.

32 Keen S. A theory of narrative empathy. *Narrative.* 2006; **14:** 207–36.

33 Halpern J. *From Detached Concern to Empathy: humanizing medical practice.* Oxford: Oxford University Press; 2001.

34 Kearny R. *On Stories.* London: Routledge; 2002.

35 Stone J. What are we all but patients? In: *Proceedings of the Third Humanism and the Healing Arts Conference.* Akron, OH: Institute for Professionalism Inquiry, Summa Health System; 2006.

36 Marci DC, Ham J, Moran E *et al.* Physiologic correlates of perceived therapist empathy and social-emotional process during psychotherapy. *J Nerv Ment Dis.* 2007; **195:** 103–11.

37 Frankel RH. Empathy for the health care professional. In: *Proceedings of the Third Humanism and Healing Arts Conference.* Akron, OH: Institute for Professionalism Inquiry, Summa Health System; 2006.

38 Wasserman RC, Inui TS, Barriatua ED *et al.* Pediatric clinicians' support for parents makes a difference: an outcome-based analysis of clinician–parent interaction. *Pediatrics.* 1984; **74:** 1047–53.

39 Ways P, Engel JD, Finkelstein P. *Clinical Clerkships: the heart of professional development.* Thousand Oaks, CA: Sage; 2000.

40 Charon R. *Narrative Medicine Workshop.* New York: Program in Narrative Medicine, College of Physicians and Surgeons, Columbia University; 2006.

41 Charon R. *Narrative Medicine: honoring the stories of illness.* New York: Oxford University Press; 2006.

42 Jones AH. Reading patients: cautions and concerns. *Lit Med.* 1994; **13:** 191–9.

43 Trautman-Banks J. The wonders of literature in medical education. In: Donnie J, editor. *The Role of the Humanities in Medical Education.* Norfolk, VA: Biomedical Ethics Program, East Virginia Medical School; 1979.

44 Daniel SL. The patient as text: a model for clinical hermeneutics. *Theor Med.* 1986; **7:** 195–210.

45 Hunter KM. Physician-writers: serving Apollo two ways at once. *Connecticut Scholar.* 1986; **8:** 27–37.

46 Terry TS, Gogel EL. Poems and patients: the balance of interpretation. *Lit Med.* 1987; **6:** 43–53.

47 Charon R. Doctor-patient/reader-writer: learning to find the text. *Soundings.* 1987; **72:** 137–52.

48 Jones AH. The color of the wallpaper. In: Charon R, Montello M, editors. *Stories Matter: the role of narrative in medical ethics.* New York: Routledge; 2002. pp. 160–63.

49 Connelly JE. The whole story. *Lit Med.* 1990; **9:** 150–61.

50 Eliot TS. *Dante,* www.quotegarden.com/poetry.html

51 Pacione A. *Rock, Paper, Poem: a learning experience,* www.poetryrepairs.com/v068.html

52 Coulehan J, Clary P. Healing the healer: poetry in palliative care. *J Palliat Med.* 2005; **8:** 382–9.

53 Gustafson MB. Methods of teaching – try haiku. *J Contin Educ Nurs.* 1979; **10:** 59–60.

54 Anthony ML. Teaching tools: nursing students and haiku. *Nurse Educ.* 1998; **23:** 14–16.

55 Lady Ise; www.ahapoetry.com/twamth1.htm

56 Hoffman Y, editor. *Japanese Death Poems.* Boston, MA: Tuttle Publishing; 1986.

57 Engel J, Pethtel L, Zarconi J. Hearing the patient's story. *Sacred Space.* 2002; **3:** 24–32.

58 Bolton G. *Reflective Practice.* London: Paul Chapman Publishing; 2001.

59 Vitz PC. The use of stories in moral development: new psychological reasons for an old educational method. *Am Psychol.* 1990; **45:** 709–20.

60 Morris DB. Narrative, ethics, and pain: thinking with stories. In: Charon R, Montello M, editors. *Stories Matter: the role of narrative in medical ethics*. New York: Routledge; 2002. pp. 196–218.

61 Frank AW. *The Wounded Storyteller*. Chicago, IL: University of Chicago Press; 1995.

62 Hensel WA, Rasco TL. Storytelling as a method for teaching values and attitudes. *Acad Med*. 1992; **67**: 500–4.

63 Murray T. What do we mean by "narrative ethics"? In: Nelson HL, editor. *Stories and Their Limits: narrative approaches to bioethics*. New York: Routledge; 1997. pp. 3–17.

64 Kearney R. *Poetics of Imagining: modern to post-modern*. New York: Fordham University Press; 1998.

65 Shapiro J, Ross V. Applications of narrative theory and therapy to the practice of family medicine. *Fam Med*. 2002; **34**: 96–100.

66 Brody H. My story is broken; can you help me fix it? *Lit Med*. 1994; **13**: 79–82.

67 Gadow S. Ethical narratives in practice. *Nurs Sci Q*. 1996; **9**: 8–9.

68 Smith DH. Telling stories as a way of doing ethics. *J Fla Med Assoc*. 1987; **74**: 581–8.

CHAPTER 7

Narrative Success and Risks of Non-Narrative Practice

> Telling stories can be healing. . . . Listening to stories also can be healing.
>
> **Dean Ornish (1: xix)**

> . . . sadly, attentive listening does not feel enough like clinical action.
>
> **Rita Charon (2: 199)**

KEY IDEAS

- Practicing narrative medicine provides connection with others through the relationships that are built between patient and caregiver.
- Listening to and caring for the patient's story offers the caregiver active participation in the relationship.
- By acting narratively, patients are encouraged to exert control over their lives and bring shared meaning to their illness.
- Practitioners benefit from intimate connection with their patients.
- Quantitative research demonstrates statistically significant positive results when narrative medicine techniques are utilized.
- The risks of not practicing narratively include less communication, less accurate information, and missed opportunities for meaningful relationships for caregiver and patient.
- Increased prevalence of malpractice litigation and decreased patient satisfaction are noted when providers do not practice narratively.
- Some patients may not want their providers to practice narrative care, but without practicing narratively, the provider will never know.

INTRODUCTION

This chapter offers judgments about the outcomes of successfully using narrative skills in clinical transactions and the risks of not using such skills for the practitioner and for the patient. Information that is used when making judgments about success and risk lies along a cognitive continuum anchored at one end by *intuitive cognition* and at the other end by *analytical cognition*. The eminent psychologist Kenneth Hammond (3, 4) has made a convincing case for such a continuum that orders various forms of cognition relative to one another. Intuition is generally taken to be an intellectual process that arrives at plausible formulations of events. Inputs to this process are generally narrative in nature – anecdotes and speculation based on close observation are typical examples. Analysis is generally taken to be an intellectual process based on logic and rationality, where the inputs are commonly quantitative and are based on some standard research process. Hammond's unique contribution with respect to a cognitive continuum is to upset the rivalry between intuition and analysis when they are set as a dichotomy, and to use the idea of a continuum to exploit the benefits of forms of cognition that lie along the continuum. Forms of cognition that lie between intuition and analysis are the most common, and include elements of both. These forms of cognition are referred to by Hammond (3) as *quasi-rationality*, a concept intended to honor the contribution of both types of cognition to making judgments about real-life events.

In this chapter we offer judgments about the efficacy of narrative practice using information at two points along the cognitive continuum – narrative accounts of success and quantitative accounts of the outcomes of narrative practices. Both types of cognitive information are empirical. Both types of information include elements of intuition and analysis. The first provides informed speculation that can contribute to our judgments (and practical knowledge) of the effects of narrative practice and at the same time suggest interesting avenues for practice and inquiry. The second provides information to inform judgments about outcomes that may be generalizable to some extent beyond particular people acting in particular clinical situations.

OUTCOMES RELATED TO NARRATIVE AND NON-NARRATIVE PRACTICE

This section is divided into two subsections. In the first, we review evidence of the potential benefits that acting in narrative ways has for patients. We categorize this evidence into that which is based on individual practitioner wisdom portrayed in narrative and speculative form, and that which is based on quantitative research. A more fine-grained analysis might be possible, but we believe that this simple categorization is practically useful for our (and your) purposes. In the second subsection, we provide a review of the potential risks of practicing in a non-narrative manner. Here, as before, we categorize these into narrative and quantitative sources.

Potential Benefits: Narrative Evidence

Pennebaker (5: 3) has observed that "When people put their emotional up-heavals into words, their physical and mental health improved markedly." Whether we use techniques involving fables, historical events, or simple open-ended questions such as asking people to talk about illness in their own terms, verbal or written expression of the story of what happened provides the background for what comes next – the actions of the patient and caregiver that facilitate healing. The process of constructing and telling the story to another, as well as listening to another's story, helps the teller and the listener to understand the experience that is being told.

Charon (2) laments in one of the opening quotes that listening to our patients tell their stories often does not feel as if we are *doing* anything to help them. We are a society of doers and problem solvers – just being mindfully present while a patient tells her story and listening attentively to the twists and turns that the story takes may not seem to be enough activity for us. Yet the benefits of encouraging the patient to speak and tell what happened and what it means is emerging (actually re-emerging) as one of the most powerful qualities of the experience between patient and caregiver.

Doing narrative practice has the potential to create a foundation for all future encounters between the patient and her physician. Creating a narrative platform for the relationship establishes what Epstein (6) describes as patient-centered communication. Narrative practice encourages the patient and the caregiver to both speak and listen, to share information in a reflective and collective manner, building a common ground from which knowledge of an illness, its treatment, and the roles that the physician and patient will play can emerge (6).

When the patient and the practitioner begin to communicate with each other through narrative practice, the foundation that is built through this communication provides the springboard for the development of their relationship. As noted in earlier discussions, this relationship-centered approach to care, if developed through a "model of mutuality" (Roter 7: 7), brings a common ground which facilitates participatory communication, deeper, more meaningful and accurate information sharing, and improved patient health outcomes. Roter (7: 13) notes that patient–caregiver encounters are ". . . visits that are facilitative in helping patients and effectively communicate their story, and express the full spectrum of concerns and questions, produce positive health outcomes." Ornish (1) agrees when he illustrates how patients who feel lonely and isolated have a higher risk of disease and premature death than patients who feel an association and connection with others.

Our culture is often described as one of loneliness, isolation, and alienation, with a loss of connectedness with other humans. Listening to and telling stories and understanding the common thread of our humanity provides a means of connecting ourselves to others and decreasing loneliness. In medical work, connectivity applies to both patient and provider. Remen (1: xxviii) writes of our current world as one of solitude, for we have become ". . . readers and watchers rather than sharers and participants." Accompanying the patient on her illness journey has the potential to provide companionship for both patient and caregiver (8, 9). The isolation felt by physicians and nurses has the potential to be alleviated for both when a fuller relationship is nurtured. Jurate Sakalys, nursing educator and researcher, describes how practicing narratively connects people and provides a reciprocal relational experience. In such an experience, the telling of and the listening to the story provide an invitation to enter another's journey, as well as an invitation for the caregiver to join the patient as the journey unfolds (10).

When a caregiver agrees to care for a patient, she is answering the patient's invitation. The answer signals the beginning of their relationship. Mattingly discusses the different roles of hero that a doctor or nurse might feel that they need to assume when answering this call, and urges caution in the following advice (11: 819):

> The relationship between patient and health professional in a caring conversation is visible in two ways: the narrative encounter itself is a relationship, and that relationship becomes a part of the patient's narrative of suffering. When a health professional enters a suffering patient's world, she or he is also entering the patient's narrative of suffering. The challenge is to do this in a way that offers sufficient hope to the patient such that the struggle to overcome obstacles becomes meaningful and bearable.

This warning should not dissuade the caregiver from engaging in a narrative relational approach to care, for it is through this relationship that the care provided and accepted by patient and practitioner becomes meaningful and bearable for both. As we saw in our discussion of the theory of complex responsive processes of relating, listening to and caring for the patient's story offers the caregiver an active rather than passive step in the care of the patient. By operating narratively, the caregiver and patient often co-construct a type of map to a complex non-linear path that helps both participants to experience more satisfying outcomes (12). Patients want, need, and seek this relationship. When faced with illness, Frank (13: 199) writes:

> ...what I wanted when I was ill, is a mutual relationship of persons who are also clinical and patient. Stories that are shared among persons can open mutual relationships; narrative reduced to clinical technique may or may not be an improvement over biomedical reductionism. When I as an ill person offer someone my story, I reach out as one human to another. Stories certainly have content; they reveal the meanings that the ill have constructed around their illnesses. But telling the story also implies a relationship that I desire with those who care for me.

Narrative practice, through the development of this relationship between the patient and the practitioner, can provide a platform for launching the formation of a more bearable illness time, and allows the patient and the caregiver a place to operate in which future decisions, plans, and actions can take place. Risdon (14) speaks of how building this relationship allows the practitioner to join our patients in a common place from which to begin. The process of compassionate presence and mindful listening to stories, the core of narrative practice as described in Chapter 6, opens a door through which the patient and practitioner walk. Once the door has been opened, both patient and practitioner have begun the work of attaching to each other within the common ground of the story. Thus begins the relationship – not a friendship of non-equals, but as Beach and colleagues (15) describe in their discussion of the principles of relationship-centered care, a relationship in which each influences the other, and where both patient and practitioner benefit.

This phase of relationship building is often the beginning of the reconstruction of the patient's life in the light of this new illness event (16–18). Frank (13) describes how through the act of telling their stories, patients are able to distance themselves from their illness and provide space to reflect on what is happening to them and how their life stories are changing. For many patients, the construction of stories around illness provides the opportunity to describe illness as part of their overall life story, rather than illness as the whole life story. Broyard (19) describes this process as constructing the illness as a character in the patient's overall story. Illness enters the patient's story in much the same way as a new character enters a play. The play changes with the introduction of the new character, but the play's title remains the same. Disease enters the patient's body, but the patient's life, although now changed through the illness, remains her life, with all of her experiences and characteristics still intact, although existentially different. Creating the conditions and encouraging patients to tell their stories provides them with opportunities to understand, maintain, or even sometimes regain control over their now changed situation. Patients are able to construct stories in which their illness plays as large or small a role in their life as they want it to play, not the size of role that the practitioner decides the illness should play.

Bury (20) describes this ability of patients to maintain or regain control over their lives as the patients' beginning steps in making meaning in the midst of the crisis that illness has produced. Greenhalgh (21) describes this meaning-making process as the time in which patients develop a contextual framework for their situation. Illness can bring dramatic change to a patient's life. Regardless of whether or not the patient is admitted to hospital, she is now in a world of foreign words, unfamiliar experiences, and often at least some degree of pain, suffering, and sorrow. Storytelling allows the patient the time and vehicle to understand this new situation, to integrate this new situation into her current lifeworld, and to begin to reconstruct this lifeworld into a new version, one within which she can successfully operate.

The following is an excerpt from a story told by a patient who was undergoing multiple treatments for cancer. She told this story in response to a question about how she was coping with cancer and all the chemotherapy and radiation that had been prescribed to combat the disease.

> I only let a little bit in every day. That way I can pace myself in what I have to deal with. When I was first diagnosed, I completely shut it all out, sort of like building a wall, really fast, around myself. And that took a lot of energy to do. Now, when I think about it, it's like I break out a piece of the wall and look through – I then decide what, on the other side of the wall, I'm going to let in and deal with on that day. Sometimes I don't let anything in. So if it seems as if I'm not paying attention to you or to what you're doing, I'm probably not because I may be having a day in which I don't want to deal with anything. I only have so much energy, you know, and I need to save it up so that I can plant my garden when I'm done with this stuff. And that's what I think about when I'm not thinking about the cancer. That, and so much more.
>
> *Anonymous*

This patient maintained control over her illness by dealing only with what she thought she could cope with at any given time. She had set her priorities, and the cancer was not high on the list. Knowing this provided me (*SAM*) with a much greater understanding of what was happening with her. She had seemed distant and uninterested. Because she would often take a little longer to answer questions or follow directions, several nurses began to describe her as non-compliant, *mentally not there*, or *a little off balance*. However, she was far from non-compliant – always on time, never missing an appointment. This patient was very much mentally there, but it was only after she told this story that we understood where she was. What could have turned out to be a progressively misunderstood care experience moved toward a relationship in which the nurses allowed her space, time, and peace, and did not demand full attention from her. In return, she began to share her garden plans and eventually her life plans with them, telling more stories and jokes, sharing recipes, and sharing parts of herself.

By practicing narratively, caregivers encourage patients to exert control and bring meaning to the illness that has entered their lives. This work often helps patients onto the path of healing. Pennebaker (2: 13) describes this progression toward healing as the patient's act of ". . . translating distress into language which ultimately allows the patient to forget, or perhaps a better phrase is to move beyond the experience of illness into a new place of healing." Risdon and Edey (14) write about how patients hunger for healing and seek authenticity in their relationships with their practitioners. This provides them with an honest space in which to begin this healing. These authors assert (14: 899):

> Patients who are ill or broken long for us to enter into authentic rela-
> tionships with them. Their hunger for healing transcends their need
> for curing. This hunger is the essence of some patients' motivation
> for relationships with alternative or complementary practitioners.
> Furthermore, medicine leaves many malnourished patients – people
> who are only partially fed by technology, accuracy, and efficiency. These
> dimensions of medicine are necessary but not sufficient for sustaining
> mind, body, and spirit. True healing and mending of brokenness is
> possible only with an authentic human relationship.

In Chapter 6, several techniques that help the caregiver to move into a more authentic relational space with the patient were described. The concept of mindfulness and the art of mindful listening were explored, for patients know when caregivers are fully present, fully engaged, and operating in an authentic relationship. The practices of mindful presence along with attentive listening provide stepping stones to authentic relationship building between patient and practitioner, and lead to healing and comfort for the patient (22, 23).

The healing power of patient stories crosses cultural, race, ethnic, and gender divisions. Saliba illustrates these powerful properties when describing how different cultures utilize storytelling in ceremonies to promote healing (24: 38–9):

> Navajo Coyote stories are used in healing rituals. They are a medicine
> intended to knit things together again after disorders have left a

wound: "in fact, to tell the stor[ies] without such moral or medicinal motives does a kind of violence to [them], and to the community. . . . In Indonesia, the shadow puppet plays provide a spiritual, learning, and healing space. . . . The purpose of these stories . . . is to draw pictures of inner thought and feeling to give an external form to the internal feeling. More specifically, it picture[s] conflict in the individual between what he want[s] to do and what he [feels] he ought to do. . . . Stories told in this kind of atmosphere, this mystically dedicated space, are healing. Not healing in an allopathic sense, which implies an illness and searches out a part of a cure, but healing in a way that allows us to see ourselves as whole. These healing stories teach us that life moves in a cosmic dance and that the balance of self-control, sacrifice, and wisdom are gifts that strengthen our spirit and hereby our mind/body. (insertions added)

In thinking about stories as a platform for connecting patients and caregivers, Fredriksson and Eriksson (12) describe this encouragement and subsequent listening and taking in of the patient's story as an interchange between patient and caregiver, as a conversation where both caringly explore the context of the conversation to find meaning in the suffering described within it. Only through exploration and attention to this suffering will the patient have a chance to move toward an eventual sense of well-being.

As a caregiver becomes the witness to this suffering, she becomes what Charon (2: 179) describes as a ". . . skilled partner in building true inter-subjectivity with sick people", and in this process healing is facilitated. As we have described in previous chapters, Charon (2) depicts this process of becoming a skilled partner as a triad of attention, representation, and affiliation. The following story illustrates this triad in action.

As a nurse, working in a busy intensive-care unit, I often had very little time to get to know my patients. The shifts were short staffed and the patients very ill, frequently intubated and unable to communicate verbally. Many days I provided care in silence, only engaging in the most cursory communication with any visitors who happened to be in the patient's room.

I often worked alongside a licensed practical nurse who had received advanced training in critical care nursing. This nurse, Carolyn, would do the *oddest* things before she entered a patient room. She would always stop and hum or sing a song before going in to care for the patient. Upon entering the patient's room, she would sit, inspect the patient completely and then talk, telling the patient who she was, what she was going to do, explaining how the patient could communicate with her, if unable to do so verbally, and what the patient could expect for the next eight hours. Then she would talk to any visitors in the room, while jotting down notes and asking many questions. Carolyn seemed to gather more information than anyone else, including the physicians caring for the patient. She wrote everything on a tablet that she kept beside the patient's chart. This tablet stayed in the room, but she was often the only person who looked at it. As she provided care for her patient, I would hear her talk about her own life, comparing her experiences to what the patient was going through. This practice of relating to the patients and their families always seemed to give Carolyn a very rich picture of her patients. No matter what the patient or family member discussed, Carolyn always had some kind of connection or common experience which seemed to draw her closer to the patient.

On one occasion, I asked Carolyn to explain her particular approach to patients. She smiled and told me that she wasn't crazy, as many people thought. She felt that it was important to clear her head every time she entered a room, because otherwise she brought a lot of stuff into the room that didn't mean anything to the patient. Singing helped her clear her head. And writing all that information down on a tablet helped her remember the *important stuff* about the patient. The chart, it seemed to her, provided no space for such information, and the *stuff* in the chart rarely helped her to take care of her patient. As for how she always had something in common with her patients, something to talk about, Carolyn smiled again and said, *We're all in this together, nobody better, nobody worse. The sooner we figure that out, the better off we'll all be.*

SAM

Carolyn knew how to become fully attentive to her patients by clearing her mind and completely focusing on being present. This is similar to the "One-Minute Mindfulness Exercise" we described in Chapter 6. She wrote down what she learned through the conversations she encouraged, knowing that these were the bits of information that would help her to provide the best care, and that they would represent the patient to her and to others who took the time to read her words. And she understood the commonality of the human condition, holding the wisdom that we are all in this together, no better or worse than anyone else.

The benefits to patients of narrative practice have been rehearsed throughout the earlier chapters, as well as in the preceding pages of this chapter. But what does the caregiver gain by practicing narratively? How does the investment in narrative practice help an already busy physician or an overworked nurse? One key answer appears to be in the power of what happens when patient and caregiver come together. This connection does not need to be perceived as all "give" on the provider's part and all "take" on the patient's part. If it is conceived deliberately, consistently, and in a nurturing way, caregivers receive as much from their connection with patients as they give, and sometimes more.

Halpern (25) warns of the *space of detached concern* in which practitioners live when they guard themselves from becoming partners with their patients, keep their patients at a distance, and decline to connect with them in other than superficial ways. Detached concern develops as a caregiver builds walls between herself and her patients, a practice that functions as a protective mechanism against the energy-draining needs and demands of her patients. This behavior is encouraged so that she will not burn out. In reality, the expense of energy necessary to build and maintain this distance may soon seal the practitioner into a place where she feels no emotion, and which may ultimately lead to greater dissatisfaction with her own career. With her humanity gone, replaced by the predictable but sterile world of technical medicine, the chances of burnout become much greater. In Chapter 6 and elsewhere we have described this phenomenon as affective blunting (26).

As we have emphasized, the techniques that develop and nurture narrative skills are not for the benefit of patients alone. Caregivers have much to gain as well. Reflective writing provides sanctuary for weary practitioners – a place to reflect on past experiences and mend past and present pain. The nurse educator and writer Vikki Holmes, writing with D Gregory (27), describes how writing a poem about the experience of caring for a patient provided the vehicle for her desire to express her feelings and emotions.

By the Sweet Bye and Bye

gentle old Welshman once a marathon runner
standing alone lost focus
wandering floundering reaching
finding us at the desk in the hall he sings
by the sweet bye and bye

lost family waiting alone for a more appropriate home
fleeting wanting goodbye he went there
returned frozen limbs sacral crevasse
still quiet a whisper of past marathons
fixed in bed 4337B

we come often with water warm hands voices blankets
weary you us and night surrender
sweet Welshman you slide away remembering we sing to you
by the sweet bye and bye.

Vikki Holmes

Holmes illustrates how her own feelings of powerlessness and hopelessness surfaced as she wrote the poem, and how through writing it she came to deepen her understanding of caring for the patient.

Holmes and Gregory describe the value of poetry reading and writing as follows (27: 1194):

> Poetry is a link with our history. It is the guardian or gatekeeper to what was rich in our past and what remains to be seen in our present and future. Poetry persuades us to attend to our personal and professional perceptions, informing us of experiences that we might otherwise

discard. In its portrait and in its permanence, poetry refuses to let nurses' experiences, feelings and images remain inconsequential, mundane or insignificant. Writing poetry is a way in which nurses can reveal the perceptions in their work and how these new-found perceptions can add depth and meaning to their practice.

In recounting the value of writing for nurses, the same could be written for the importance of writing to the experiences of all caregivers. We should not be afraid to "fall into" our patients as noted by Broyard (28), for it is the act of maintaining distance that impedes our own growth and healing.

Potential Benefits: Quantitative Evidence

Just as the narrative evidence for the benefits of narrative practice continues to grow, the wealth of analytic evidence addressing these same benefits has also begun to accumulate. Although there have been few studies of the direct impact of narrative practice per se, a number of elements of this form of practice – for example, reflective writing, empathic communication, and relationship-centered care – have demonstrated meaningful benefits.

Pennebaker (2) cites the demonstration of positive effects on blood markers of immune function and lower incidence of depression when patients participated in writing exercises similar to those described in Chapter 6. Smyth and colleagues (29) noted that when patients with asthma or rheumatoid arthritis wrote about stressful events in their lives, they experienced improved health status. They found that the asthma patients who participated in these writing exercises showed improved lung function and the arthritis patients showed improved disease activity compared with control groups.

Trummer and colleagues (30) described their findings for a group of 99 cardiac patients, who experienced a 1-day decrease in length of hospitalization time compared with the 100 cardiac patients in the control group, a 15% decrease in post-surgery tachyarrhythmia compared with the control group, faster transfer to less intensive-care beds post-operatively than occurred in the control group, and higher post-hospital patient satisfaction score when cared for by physicians and nurses who had recently undergone intensive training in narrative medicine techniques aimed at improving communication skills.

By improving communication between patients and physicians, Roter and Hall (31) also demonstrated improved patient satisfaction leading to improved patient compliance with medical treatments. Findings from their research into educating students and practicing physicians in the areas of empathic communication skills also demonstrated the ability of these practitioners to practice in a more narrative way, which in turn enhanced patient conversations, improved patient adherence to treatment regimens, and increased patient satisfaction. Rogers and colleagues (32) demonstrated similar findings in a London-based study in which palliative care patients noted that the greatest dissatisfaction with the hospital care they received was centered on their own and their family's perception of dehumanization. They stated that they often felt that the nurse–patient relationship had broken down. Rogers and colleagues summarize their findings as follows (32: 772):

> As such, the causes of dissatisfaction for this particular group of patients may be seen as very similar to the causes of dissatisfaction with health care in general. Our findings suggest that people's expectations of care during the last years of life differ very little from expectations of health care in general.

As noted above, all patients – whether they are in the process of preparing to live or to die – want the same attentive, empathic, relationship-oriented care. They want to be able to express their pain, find comfort in the companionship of their caregivers, and move toward a place where they may heal.

Potential Risks: Narrative Evidence

The benefits of narrative practice for patient and caregiver are many. What happens when health care providers practice non-narratively? Are there risks they take that could lead to potential problems for their patients and themselves? If the reverse of the previously explored benefits is assumed, patients would not participate in the relationship-centered approach to care that Frank (13), Roter (7), Beach (15) and others demonstrated as being at the core of what patients want and need. Not practicing within a narrative context also affects the practitioner, for as Charon (33: 1897) writes, the physician who does not practice narratively does not:

> ... reach and join their patients in illness, recognize their own personal journeys through medicine, acknowledge kinship with and duties toward other health care professionals, and inaugurate consequential discourse with the public about health care.

Epstein (6) maintains that when physicians learn attentiveness and curiosity in developing their listening skills, they are able to improve communication between themselves and their patients and subsequently improve their diagnostic accuracy due to the increased information that they receive through practicing these skills. Without this attention and probing with genuine curiosity, caregivers miss the clues that patients give, assumptions replace true knowledge, and actions are based on assumptions rather than on truth.

Is it fair to say that not all patients are worthy of narrative practice? This again is based on an assumption that needs a warning label. Even what some would describe as a mundane, boring patient has a story to be shared if someone is willing to take the time to ask, as evidenced by the following excerpt of a story told by Faith Fitzgerald, a practicing internist (34: 11–12):

When I was a young attending at San Francisco General Hospital, morning rounds usually consisted of briefly going over the 15 or 20 patients admitted to the team the night before and then concentrating on the "interesting" ones. I was righteous and was determined to teach the house staff that there were no uninteresting patients, so I asked the resident to pick the dullest one.

He chose an old woman admitted out of compassion because she had been evicted from her apartment and had nowhere else to go. She had no real medical history, but was simply suffering from the depredations of antiquity and abandonment. I led the protesting group of house staff to her bedside. She was monosyllabic in her responses and gave a history of no substantive content. Nothing, it seemed, had ever really happened to her. She had lived a singularly unexciting life as a hotel maid. She could not even (or would not) tell stories of famous people caught in her hotel in awkward situations. I was getting desperate, as it did seem that this woman was truly uninteresting. Finally, I asked her how long she had lived in San Francisco.

Years and years, she said.

Was she here for the earthquake?

No, she came after.

Where did she come from?

Ireland.

When did she come?

1912.

Had she ever been to a hospital before?

Once.

How did that happen?

Well, she had broken her arm.

How had she broken her arm?

A trunk fell on it.

A trunk?

Yes.

What kind of trunk?

A steamer trunk.

How did that happen?

The boat lurched.

The boat?

The boat that was carrying her to America.

Why did the boat lurch?

It hit the iceberg.

Oh! What was the name of the boat?

The *Titanic*.

Faith Fitzgerald

This patient had been a passenger on the *Titanic*, and through the discovery of her narrative she became extraordinary. But she was always extraordinary. Patients like this one – indeed potentially all patients – expose their extraordinariness through the sharing of their stories.

Potential Risks: Quantitative Evidence

Research on the conditions associated with malpractice suits suggests that there is a decrease in the number of malpractice suits brought to court from patients who benefited from narrative practice. As noted in a review of research conducted by Freeborn, Levinson, and Mullooly (35), several studies documented significantly less litigation when patients perceived their physicians as being empathic and demonstrating attentive communication skills essential to narrative clinical work. Kielhorn (36) cites research connecting forms of communication with patients' decisions to file malpractice claims. Patients who perceived their physicians as open to discussions and willing to include them in care decisions were less likely to sue. Nakajima and Bidaillon (37) report similar findings, and note that 12% of total claims reviewed in their study involved communication failures as the central risk management issue. Another study, by Levinson and colleagues, which compared the communication habits of surgeons and primary care physicians, noted the following findings (38: 556):

> [a study of] communication behaviors associated with physician malpractice history found that physician–patient communication for primary care physicians with prior malpractice claims differs from that of those without a claims history. In comparison with their peers who had at least two claims, primary care physicians without a claims history provided patients with more information about what to expect and, in the course of the visit, laughed and used humor more frequently. They were also more likely to solicit patients' opinions, to check their level of understanding, and to encourage them to talk. In addition, primary care physicians without claims spent more time in routine visits than their peers with claims.

It can be argued that narrative practice promotes richer and deeper forms of personal and empathic communication. So these studies suggest that practicing without narrative competence is potentially damaging for those who seek engaged relationships with their caregivers.

BARRIERS TO NARRATIVE PRACTICE, AND CAUTIONARY TALES

Given what is known about the benefits of narrative practice and the risks we run when we do not develop and refine our narrative skills, are there times when practicing narratively is not possible? Are there barriers that prevent us from developing our moral imagining skills, reading our patients' narratives closely, or being mindfully present for our patients? Are there patients who do not want (or who will not accept) our attempts to listen attentively to their stories, will not allow us to use our curiosity to its fullest, and do not want us to know who they really are?

If we have never actively explored the lived experiences of others, as we can do, for example, by reading the writings of authors such as Frank (13), Kleinman (39), Charon (2), or Remen (1), we may never experience the possibilities of what living in another's narrative world could bring to our understanding of who they are and who we are. If we do not take the time to learn how to be mindfully present to our patients as discussed by Connelly (22), or appreciate what Halpern (25) is telling us when she cautions us about what happens when we shut off our patients and eventually ourselves from our work, we may become emotionally detached and empty. If we never learn the value of reading the poetry of writers like Davis and Schaefer (40) or Stone (41), we may never appreciate how often poetry speaks in metaphor just as patients do. Without role models, peers, mentors, and people who support our narrative work and help narrative novices to find the theory, background, and stories to assist their development into competent narrative practitioners, we may fail to move toward a narratively competent system of care – a system that many of our patients want and all of them deserve. There are barriers to this work. However, if each of us accepts the responsibility to teach, to lead by example, to study the best role models and practices, and to disseminate their work and results, we can change the way that health care is provided.

It should also be recognized that there are some patients who do not want us in their narrative, and who are not willing to share their stories with us. Swenson and colleagues (42) have reported that in a study of patient preferences for patient-centered or biomedical communication styles, nearly one-third of the patients preferred a non-patient-centered, authoritarian, biomedical style of communication and health care delivery. Levinson and colleagues (43), in a national study of public preferences, similarly found that not all patients want to participate in decision making about their health care. Furthermore, in a review of patient experiences and interviews, Quill and Brody state (44: 64):

> Sharing of information is presumed to be "patient centered" because experts presume that patients want it, patients generally say that they want it, and it can enable patients to participate more actively in medical decisions. Offering patients choices is also thought to be a good thing, but may not be sufficient to address the needs of patients who want a clear physician recommendation. Some patients might perceive "authoritarian" communication styles, not generally regarded as patient-centered, as caring and involved.

These studies suggest that patients under certain circumstances consider a meaningful relationship with their caregiver to be defined in strictly technical ways. Such patients are often relatively healthy, may be described as the "worried well", or may have conditions that are neither serious nor life-threatening. In these situations, such patients seek a more mechanical approach to treatment.

We should recognize that all patients come to us with unique needs and expectations. The communication style and the form of relationship that work with one patient may not work well with the next one. This is where the caregiver's virtue of wisdom (phronesis) comes into play. Being competent in a variety of narrative and biomedical skills, the wise caregiver understands how to balance these approaches for the benefit of her patient, while recognizing that her patient's circumstances and corresponding needs shift over time. It follows that the patient as an individual brings her history, her culture, and her life experience to the examination table. This mixture of so many features makes the patient who she is, and this is where we as caregivers need to meet her. The following story concerns a patient who, because of her background, culture, experience, and gender did not want to participate in any collaborative attempts to resolve her medical problems.

Mrs S, an older Italian woman with beautiful white hair pulled up in a bun and smooth olive skin comes to see her physician for quarterly assessments of her hypertension. During each visit she sits silently, smiling politely while her doctor reviews the blood pressure readings and talks about her medication regimen. As the nurse I measured her blood pressure, weight, and temperature in preparation for her encounter with the physician. Mrs S. never speaks to me, only smiles politely, the same as she does with the doctor. Years go by, and the same routine occurs. Mrs S. never misses an appointment, is always on time, always takes her medication, and always does exactly what she is told to do, never asking any questions, never revealing anything about what she is thinking or feeling.

Finally, one day as I recorded her latest vital signs, I asked her why she never asked any questions of me or her doctor. I couldn't understand why she wouldn't share any of her life with me. What was she hiding? Why didn't she cooperate? She looked at me with wide eyes and an almost stunned, scared expression on her face, and didn't reply. Again I asked her why she had no questions. This time she took a deep breath and slowly responded, "Why would I have questions? I know nothing about this. That is why I pay the doctor. I would insult him if I asked a question. It would be like I was questioning his knowledge or your knowledge as well. You are both educated – I would never insult you with a question."

I tried to explain that we would not be insulted and that we would welcome her questions, encouraging her to share in the conversation about her health.

She did not speak again, but merely smiled politely, looking past me as she awaited her turn with her doctor.

SAM

This was a patient who was neither willing nor able to participate in patient-centered, narrative care. Her world was structured by a culture of unquestioning respect for authority and medical expertise. To ask questions, talk about herself, and move into a space where she might be on an equal plane with her caregivers was inconceivable to her. Mrs S was content to follow her doctor's orders, and not only expected but actually preferred a paternalistic approach to her care.

Some patients do not wish to operate in a narrative world. Trying to force them into this approach would be a great disservice to their personhood. However, this is where we need to raise a cautionary flag. The caution enters when we ask how we know that a patient does not want to participate as an equal partner and/or cannot partake narratively. Do we assume, because a patient remains silent through encounter after encounter, that they do not want to be a partner in the care process? Or is it necessary, as with a clinical diagnosis, to rule out other possible explanations for the silence? Without the moral imagination to inquire, I (SAM) might never have understood the world in which Mrs S was raised and in which she had lived for many decades. Without the skills of attentive listening and mindful presence, her physician might never have understood how, through her silence and polite smiles, Mrs S was sharing as much about herself as she could. Finally, without the practice of reflective writing, I as the nurse who participated in her care would not have written the story of Mrs S – a story that preserved her uniqueness and humanity, and that strengthened my ability to bear witness and learn from her and hopefully teach others.

FURTHER ACTIVITIES

1   Readers who are interested in learning more about the benefits of practicing narrative medicine are encouraged to consult the following texts and articles:
    - Kleinman A. *The Illness Narratives: suffering, healing and the human condition.* New York: Basic Books; 1988.
    - Pennebaker JW. Telling stories: the health benefits of narrative. *Lit Med.* 2006; **19:** 3–18.
    - Greenhalgh T. *What Seems to be the Trouble? Stories in illness and healthcare.* Oxford: Radcliffe Publishing; 2006.
    - Sakalys J. Restoring the patient's voice: the therapeutics of illness narratives. *J Holist Nurs.* 2003; **21:** 228–41.
    - Roter DL, Hall JA. *Doctors Talking with Patients/Patients Talking with Doctors: improving communication in medical visits.* 2nd ed. Westport, CT: Praeger; 2006.
2   In addition, the following websites contain useful information on personal experiences of health and illness from the viewpoint of patients and clinicians:
    - www.dipex.org.uk
    - www.patientvoices.org.uk

REFERENCES

1 Ornish D. Foreword. In: Remen RN. *Kitchen Table Wisdom.* New York: Riverhead Books; 1996. p. xix.

2 Charon R. *Narrative Medicine: honoring the stories of illness.* New York: Oxford University Press; 2006.

3 Hammond KR. *Human Judgment and Social Policy: irreducible uncertainty, inevitable error, and unavoidable injustice.* New York: Oxford University Press; 1996.

4 Hammond KR. *Judgments Under Stress.* New York: Oxford University Press; 2000.

5 Pennebaker JW. Telling stories: the health benefits of narrative. *Lit Med.* 2000; **19:** 3–18.

6 Epstein RM. Making communication research matter: what do patients notice, what do patients want, and what do patients need? *Patient Educ Couns.* 2006; **60:** 272–8.

7 Roter D. The enduring and evolving nature of the patient–physician relationship. *Patient Educ Couns.* 2000; **39:** 5–15.

8 Shapiro J. The use of narrative in the doctor–patient encounter. *Fam Syst Med.* 1993; **11:** 7–53.

9 Taylor C. Narrating practice: reflective accounts and the textual construction of reality. *J Adv Nurs.* 2003; **42:** 244–51.

10 Sakalys JA. Restoring the patient's voice: the therapeutics of illness narratives. *J Holist Nurs.* 2003; **21:** 228–41.

11 Mattingly C. The concept of therapeutic 'emplotment.' *Soc Sci Med.* 1994; **38:** 811–22.

12 Fredriksson L, Eriksson K. The patient's narrative of suffering: a path to health? *Scand J Caring Sci.* 2001; **15:** 3–11.

13 Frank A. Just listening: narrative and deep illness. *Fam Syst Health.* 1998; **16:** 197–212.

14 Risdon C, Edey L. Human doctoring: bringing authenticity to our care. *Acad Med.* 1999; **74:** 896–9.

15 Beach MC, Inui T, Frankel R *et al.* Relationship-centered care: a constructive reframing. *J Gen Intern Med.* 2006; **21:** S3–8.

16 Rimmon-Kenan S. The story of "I": illness and narrative identity. *Narrative.* 2002; **10:** 9–27.

17 Eggly S. Physician–patient co-construction of illness narratives in the medical interview. *Health Commun.* 2002; **14:** 339–60.

18 Brody H. "My story is broken; can you help me fix it?" Medical ethics and the joint construction of narrative. *Lit Med.* 1994; **13:** 79–92.

19 Broyard A. *Intoxicated by my Illness and Other Writing on Life and Death.* New York: Fawcett Columbine; 1993.

20 Bury M. Illness narratives: fact or fiction? *Sociol Health Illn.* 2001; **23:** 263–85.

21 Greenhalgh T. *What Seems To Be The Trouble? Stories in illness and healthcare.* Oxford: Radcliffe Publishing; 2006.

22 Connelly JE. Narrative possibilities: using mindfulness in clinical practice. *Perspect Biol Med.* 2005; **48:** 84–94.

23 Charon R. Narrative medicine: attention, representation, affiliation. *Narrative.* 2005; **13:** 261–70.

24 Saliba M. Story language: a sacred healing space. *Lit Med.* 2000; **19:** 38–50.

25 Halpern J. *From Detached Concern to Empathy: humanizing medical practice.* New York: Oxford University Press; 2001.

26 Ways P, Engel JD, Finkelstein P. *Clinical Clerkships: the heart of professional development.* Thousand Oaks, CA: Sage; 2000.

27 Holmes V, Gregory D. Writing poetry: a way of knowing nursing. *J Adv Nurs.* 1998; **28:** 1191–4.

28 Broyard A. Doctor, talk to me. *New York Times Magazine,* 26 August 1990, p. 33.

29 Smyth JM, Stone AA, Hurewitz A *et al.* Effects of writing about stressful experiences on symptom reduction in patients with asthma or rheumatoid arthritis. *JAMA.* 1999; **281:** 1304–9.

30 Trummer UF, Mueller UO, Nowak P *et al.* Does physician–patient communication that aims at empowering patients improve clinical outcome? A case study. *Patient Educ Couns.* 2006; **61:** 299–306.

31 Roter DL, Hall JA. *Doctors Talking with Patients/Patients Talking with Doctors: improving communication in medical visits.* Westport, CT: Praeger; 2006.

32 Rogers A, Karlsen S, Addington-Hall J. Issues and innovations in nursing practice. *J Adv Nurs.* 2000; **3:** 768–74.

33 Charon R. Narrative medicine: a model for empathy, reflection, profession, and trust. *JAMA.* 2001; **286:** 1897–902.

34 LaCombe MA, editor. *On Being a Doctor 2.* Philadelphia, PA: American College of Physicians; 2000.

35 Freeborn DK, Levinson W, Mullooly JP. Medical malpractice and its consequences: does physician gender play a role? *Journal Gender Cult Health.* 1999; **4:** 201.

36 Kielhorn TM. Reducing risk by improving communication. *Permanente J.* 1997; **1:** 69–70.

37 Nakajimi K, Bidaillon D. Communication issues in the managed care environment. *Forum.* 1996; **17:** 6–9.

38 Levinson W, Rober Dl, Mullooly JP *et al.* Physician–patient communication: the relationship with malpractice claims among primary care physicians and surgeons. *JAMA.* 1977; **277:** 553–9.

39 Kleinman A. *The Illness Narratives: suffering, healing and the human condition.* New York: Basic Books; 1988.

40 Davis C, Schaefer J. *Between the Heartbeats: poetry and prose by nurses.* Iowa City, IA: University of Iowa Press; 1995.

41 Stone J. *Music from Apartment 8: new and selected poems.* Baton Rouge, LA: Louisiana State University Press; 2004.

42 Swenson SL, Zattler P, Lo B. 'She gave it her best shot right away': patient experiences of biomedical and patient-centered communication. *Patient Educ Couns.* 2006; **61:** 200–11.

43 Levinson W, Kao A, Kuby A *et al.* Not all patients want to participate in decision making: a national study of public preferences. *J Gen Intern Med.* 2005; **20:** 531–5.

44 Quill TE, Brody H. Physician recommendations and patient autonomy: finding a balance between physician power and patient choice. *Ann Intern Med.* 1996; **125:** 63–9.

PART 4

Personal Perspectives on Narrative in Health Care

Part 4 concludes the book with conversations recorded with several nurses and physicians, all of whom practice narratively. In addition, several of these practitioners have been key figures in the development of narrative approaches to health care. As you read their responses to the same set of questions, you will witness the rich diversity of thought and the deep passion among these professionals.

CHAPTER 8

Conversations with Practitioners

We conclude the book with a set of conversations carried out with eight health care clinicians who purposively honor the stories of their patients and profession. Four conversations are with physicians: **V**alerie **G**ilchrist (family physician); **R**ita **C**haron (general internist and literary scholar); **J**ack **C**oulehan (family physician and poet); and **T**homas **B**oniface (orthopedic surgeon). Three conversations are with nurses: **C**ourtney **D**avis (nurse practitioner and poet); **E**arl **M**cFarland (cardiology nurse practitioner); and **J**udy **S**chaefer (nurse and poet). Several of these clinicians (Charon, Coulehan, Davis, and Schaefer) have contributed significant scholarly work to the field of narrative health care.

Each conversation lasted from 45 to 90 minutes and was guided by a set of open-ended questions clustered into four broad themes:
- important characteristics of narrative medicine
- conditions that have prompted a narrative movement
- the relationship between narrative medicine and other related movements
- reactions to some frequently mentioned issues associated with narrative practice.

The conversations were tape recorded, transcribed, and provided to the interviewees.

This chapter is organized according to the questions that were asked, with responses from the interviewees. To make these extensive interviews manageable within the limited space in this chapter, we have selected a subset of the questions and have included a selection of responses from the physicians and nurses. In selecting responses, we have tried to include a diversity of viewpoints. When a response echoed sentiments similar to those of other respondents, only the more detailed response was recorded here. The conversations have been edited for narrative flow, but neither substance nor voice has been altered.

The complete set of questions may be found at www.summahealth.org (in "Find It", type "Institute for Professionalism Inquiry"). We encourage you to participate in the conversation by adding your thoughts to any or all of these questions.

IMPORTANT CHARACTERISTICS OF NARRATIVE MEDICINE

Interviewer (I): What do you see as important characteristics of narrative medicine?

RC: I don't think it's simply a matter of patients telling their illness story. I think that's part of it. I think that's not the whole thing. I'm not sure what "narrative-based" means . . . I think that "narrative-based", as an adjective, was used initially as a retort . . . to evidence-based medicine. . . . I don't see there's particular usefulness in pitting narrative against evidence. . . . [our] program has partnered up with the Columbia group committed to evidence-based medicine, led by an internist emergency medicine physician . . . and very, very engaged in the evidence-based medicine field. . . . He came to us to say, "evidence-based medicine lacks what you in narrative medicine know." I was able to say to him "Narrative medicine lacks what you in evidence-based medicine know." So we have formed a joint intensive study seminar. We call it narrative–evidence-based medicine, realizing that there is evidence to be had in narrative. . . . So, to dichotomize those two seems a mistake to me, and seems to relinquish a lot of what I believe is salient to clinical practice, which is to say narrative-based medicine, by definition, is not meant to point to medicine that does not have evidence. . . . We're at a point in this field already of high complexity.

JC: I think the most important characteristic is that it is another attempt to bring us back to the story of the patient as central to medical practice. So the use of the construct of narrative, the whole movement around that, is another way of refocusing us. Beyond that, some aspects of the movement are relatively new; for example, the use of narrative by trainees and others to enhance their self-awareness, and the use of narrative in teaching about different aspects of patients' understanding of their world.

CD: Ideally, narrative-based medicine provides an opportunity for caregivers to pay more attention to, and give more recognition to, the patient's point of view. If a caregiver practices narrative-based medicine, that's a good indication that he or she is willing not only to suppress the desire to be "right" – to come to a diagnosis quickly – but also to spend time talking with and listening to patients.

Narrative-based medicine also helps us acknowledge that the relationship between patient and caregiver is a social relationship – not the same kind of social relationship we might have outside the hospital, but an important and unique relationship in the patient's life and in the provider's life as well. I think, in a sense, narrative-based medicine "levels the playing field", particularly when the caregiver sits down, puts aside the chart and the pen and really attends to what the patient is saying, both in word and in implication – this gives the patient's narrative as much authority as the provider's.

Perhaps for me the most important characteristic of narrative-based medicine is that it provides the patient with a benevolent witness to his or her story. Depending on the caregiver, this focused way of listening and communicating may lead to more holistic, personalized care. That is, if it really works. I say this because I'm very aware, personally, of having one foot in the literature and medicine world – where we talk in seminars and workshops about how to use novels and poetry to enhance our ability to give compassionate patient care – and another foot in the trenches – the busy clinic where time and insurance too often dictate how we actually deliver care. In our seminars, we're able to take time and reflect: the patient has a story; the family has a story; the caregiver has a story. We look at these stories and dissect them, understanding how essential this is and how wonderful. But, when I go back to work, I don't see many caregivers practicing narrative-based medicine. I don't see the doctors I work with engaged in compassionate listening. I don't see the residents using narrative techniques or even having the slightest interest in doing so.

TB: I think of the important characteristics as being those where you actually consider the patient's story or history first, perhaps foremost, rather than looking at the test results or the numbers. I've seen a gradual shift, both on the part of physicians and on the part of patients, to start with: Did you see my MRI? Or what does my MRI show? Or how's my blood pressure today? Or how's my cholesterol? Numbers and tests have assumed a greater sense of emphasis, whereas narrative medicine is the opposite. It is really based on: What's your history? What do you feel? What's happening? How are you doing? How is your life going? It is more historical or story-based, tuned more to the patient and their problems.

I: What do you think the patient gains from telling her illness story? And what does the physician or nurse gain by attending fully?
VG: Two things. First of all, I immediately flash back to the legitimization of whatever they present with . . . an example being victims of domestic violence . . . when they tell that story, it legitimizes that this is a story of value and therefore legitimizes them in that story. So that's one piece. The other piece that the patient gains is the reframing of the story. Every time you tell that story . . . you have different understandings. As we try and understand the implicit or explicit "why" and relationships of the various components either within oneself or with oneself to whatever context there is, whether it be family or situation. . . . So, it's the reframing.

What does the physician gain? The immediate phrase that jumps to mind was what Ian McWhinney called "the acquaintance with the particulars." That's what it meant to me . . . the knowing of that particular patient in a very different way. So the physician gains understanding. . . . Also there's a wealth of material that helps you be a better physician, in terms of making the right diagnoses, in terms of what will be more or less helpful for this particular patient. . . . I think that beyond that for me personally, there's a human component that resonates at the heart of what I love about interacting with other human beings. It's that piece that is much more at a non-intellectual level that is fulfilling for me. As another individual . . . I'm continually moved by other people. That sense of having known somebody at a non-superficial level just makes me feel more human.

RC: Well, it's not as if it's a thing easily done, that has gains and losses. . . . The ill person is indeed more than one subject and . . . there is more than one story to be accounted for. So, [for] anybody who's ill, the telling of the so-called "story" is what goes on throughout the whole "kit and caboodle." It's not that "I was well, then I got sick, then I was better" or even "My migraines come when the weather changes or when I get my period or especially if I have too much alcohol, and then I have to stay in bed for two days with the lights out, and then I vomit." . . . Then there's the bigger story about, where did your migraines come from? Or how do your migraines help you? Or what do your migraines cost you? Or who do your migraines bind you to? Or who do your migraines free you from? All of those kinds of questions are, if you will, different rooms of this account, this narrative. So I don't want to mislead anybody into thinking "Oh, I got the story; next, on to the EKG."

JC: The first thing . . . is that we have to begin with the fact that the central feature, or at least a primary feature, of the student's/trainee's/doctor's ability to elicit the patient's story and to understand the patient, is to get the primary data of the illness. By using a narrative-based approach, you obtain more clinically useful data. . . . You're able to diagnose the situation as well as the illness, better able to tailor your intervention, whatever it might be, and to ensure a better relationship. I want to emphasize that we're not talking simply about aspects of understanding the patient – cultural, social, personal style, etc. We're really also talking about getting more accurate biomedical information . . . in so far as the physician's job is to benefit the patient, then the physician hopes to gain the ability to make better judgments. I think there's a sense in which narrative medicine is more efficient. Again, if you look at efficiency as getting to the bottom of things in the most direct fashion, being able to help the patient, let's say, in the most efficient way, then I would argue that the narrative approach to medicine is more efficient than a mechanical approach. The other thing, of course, is that the doctor also benefits. You have the opportunity of learning more about yourself and your own story, your own interaction with the patient. In so far as you can do this, you avoid many of the emotional problems that occur with doctors, in terms of depression, stress, burnout, and so forth. There is a sort of a positive feedback loop, in the sense that once the doctor becomes reflective about his or her own approaches and needs and reactions to situations, then the narrative in patient care helps the doctor by allowing her or him to use the outcome – being a more reflective person – in a way that it becomes a positive feedback loop.

CD: I think when patients are encouraged to tell their stories, this "telling" gives them a chance to review their own histories and, in particular, the history of their current illness. This review may help them to discover some new emotional truths about their lives and their interactions with others, including their families. It may help them to understand or fully experience their illnesses. Patients often don't get a chance to be heard, non-judgmentally, in the "traditional" patient–caregiver encounter. In the traditional encounter the patient might mention a few symptoms and suddenly the doctor or caregiver might be talking, interrupting, having already made some tentative diagnosis. For one thing, the practice of narrative-based medicine gives the patient a chance to talk as much as the caregiver! I think it also gives the patient a chance to create a statement, a history, a biography, a re-counting of his or her life, as well as of the illness that has come into that life. Being able to tell their story and to be fully heard also gives patients a chance to see their illness as not separate from their lives but part of their lives.

I can tell you what I've gained from my experiences. First, I find there's a deep emotional satisfaction in just being present with a patient in a very human and intimate way – knowing that I've shared a space and time with someone who is unique, someone who is in a strange environment and probably truly frightened. For me, attending fully to a patient helps to lessen the more deadening aspects of caregiving – the sorrows, the losses, the demands of time, the required but too often overwhelming paperwork.

TB: Well, the story, containing words more than numbers . . . would include psychological issues, emotional issues, societal issues, family, and how you feel about everything. A lot of what we do in medicine, particularly my being an orthopedist . . . has to do with pain. . . . It doesn't show up on a lab test or a scale or X-ray, so what the patient gains is a more full expression of what they feel. The emotional side is part of it. For me, the importance of this is that the patient telling a story is really the uniquely human aspect.

I think it follows that the physician gains an ability to treat the patient as a whole person, to treat all the facets of the disease or at least be involved in it. If we can't fix everything, we can at least include it in the treatment. We can understand how somebody feels about their illness or their disability, about their problem. We can help them to deal with that aspect. . . . I think it's important that the physician gains the ability to help the patient on those things we can't solve, to get them to digest the process and accept whatever they have that we might not be able to fully address. . . . I think [the physician] can gain more full appreciation of the human condition. The fascinating thing to me is that it's an honor to be invited into somebody's life at that level. I think the physician gains a sense of satisfaction that they're working at that level in the relationship . . .

EM: I look at patients as being fragile and isolated. . . . [they] can't speak to members of their family because they're trying to protect them from the problems that they're going through, they don't want them to feel their pain. Even if you're surrounded by loved ones, you still can be extremely isolated.

When I'm with a patient and I'm listening to them and speaking with them, I feel this sense of isolation is lessened if not dissolved altogether. . . . I sometimes feel like I'm the one person that they can talk to about all the things that they're going through – all the suffering. That to me is the most important part, from the patient's point of view. We develop a partnership, a healing relationship that develops over time. Trusting is part of the narrative.

From the caregiver's point of view it helps me when we talk in depth and I listen in depth. It helps to get a clear picture of that whole person. I can provide better care for them because I understand all of the ramifications of their illness. I feel better about our relationship myself. I learn about myself as I'm learning about them. . . . It just re-affirms to me the humanity of both of us. . . . That is a very rewarding thing for me. It keeps me doing what I want to do.

JS: Storytelling is a healing process. I think it's healing for the patient. I think it's healing for the practitioner. Pulling the elements of your story together is very gratifying. It's satisfying at a core human level.

I: How has your narrative competence changed your practice?
VG: . . . it's changed my work as a teacher and an administrator. So the same characteristics of relating to people that you carry into a clinical encounter I think you carry into an administrative role and into a teaching role. . . . You take narrative competence or narrative perspective into your teaching, because as somebody presents . . . whatever . . . pain . . . or headaches or hypertension . . . I end up saying, at least once, if not more, "tell me about this person." Who is she? Is she married? Who's at home? What work does she do? . . . In essence, tell me their story. So that's one level that enters your teaching.

RC: Well, indeed it has alerted me . . . to not get in the way of telling . . . I'm beginning to know how varied are the means of the so-called telling. . . . The more we do this work, the more we're impressed with the enactment of these accounts. They're not just spoken words in a few paragraphs from a speaker to a listener. . . . Something might start if you ask someone, "Tell me what I, as your doctor, should know about your situation", which I've found is as decent a way to invite your story as any. I know I'm going to hear bits of it for the next 20 years. My training, as an internist, lets me know things about my tellers, in part, before they know it, at least I can guess things. . . . I'm more curious than I had been earlier as a doctor, far more "on the edge of my seat" saying "what's going to happen today?" It's a different kind of thrill.

. . . one result of my increasing narrative competence was to realize that much of what goes on in the office visit – routine, typical, general internist, 20-minute visit – was lost to me because I couldn't see it all. I couldn't take it all in, especially because I was participating in it. I understood that there was much more going on that I was squandering. So I started . . . a witness project and I hired good observers and good writers to sit with me, in the office, as I see patients. . . . Patients all say "sure it's fine that she sits in." . . . I want people who are not clinicians because they wouldn't be blinded to the same thing I am. . . . I ask them to take field notes, as would an anthropologist, not about the technical business, but about what they "see." . . . she [the witness] wrote Chekhovian representations of the visit. She would give them to me at the end of the day. She wouldn't write about every patient, maybe two or three, and they would be rather extensive, highly naturalistic, descriptive prose about the conversation, about the appearance of the patient, the behavior of the patient, and the behavior of me. Much of it was very humbling for me because my witness is honest and brave and knows that I want a fair representation of what happens.

I wanted the patient to have a record of our visit, too. I had been in the habit of giving the patient a print-out of what I wrote in the clinic notes. But I took that more seriously, especially as I started to read the witness field notes, because I could see how much was going on that I wasn't really paying attention to. Knowing that I give the patient a copy of his or her clinic note, and this goes online, so this is available to any other doctor, nurse, or social worker in the hospital, I started writing it in a way that the patient would understand. It wasn't abbreviations and numbers – it was in words that the patient would understand. . . . So the narrative competence, in a funny way, has had these big ramifications because now everybody in the hospital knows these things. When one of my patients shows up in the emergency room and they open up [the chart], they know the patient has gone through a profound significant loss because the cat died or because the common-law wife died or because the apartment was broken into or whatever the case may be.

JC: I would say that my whole medical practice over 30 some years has been a maturation process in terms of understanding myself better. . . . From the very beginning, I was more interested in narrative. . . . What has probably changed over time is that, as I have practiced in different settings at different times, I've learned from the different external constraints on my time and different populations of patients. I guess I've learned to be more versatile and open . . .

CD: I think that from the time I became a nurse, my intuitive instinct was to listen to my patients' stories, long before I knew anything about narrative-based medicine. . . . So I've been listening to the patient's narrative all along.

Also, as a writer, I've learned how to read literature on two levels – on the surface and on a deeper, metaphorical level. That has taught me to listen to a patient's story in the same way, aware of the spoken words, the metaphors and similes, and the body language. I was working as a nurse at the same time that I was becoming a writer. Those two paths didn't come together for a long time, but I think they were feeding each other all along. Because I could "suspend belief" in writing poems, I could also suspend belief when I was with a patient, meaning that I could be open to any apparent conflicts either in the patient's life or in the patient's story. This openness helped me, still helps me, to be aware and accepting of the profound and moving moments that occur when I'm in an exam room with a patient. And so although I was practicing narrative-based nursing already, learning and exploring more about narrative-based medicine has made me extremely aware of – and more careful about – my interactions with patients, how writing informs my caregiving and how caregiving informs my writing.

TB: I think I've been using narrative medicine, but in a sort of naive way. . . . I think it's expanded my scope of treatment, my ability to treat people. I'm a surgeon, and yet I'm finding I'm treating people as successfully as before, or maybe more successfully without surgery than with surgery because their problems are not all anatomical or structural. It's helped me to look into the story more and really help people get through their problems without having to do something like surgery. It's one of the aspects of care that I think goes beyond the technical expertise to arrive at a plan, and how to use therapy. It's a broader type of care I can provide, not just doing surgery.

I: What are the risks you see in a narrative practice?
VG: The major risk for me is that I get sucked in. I could spend half an hour or 45 minutes with every patient and the story. . . . Then I would be even further behind than I usually am. So it's timing.

RC: The risk you see is maybe you think you know more than you do. It's easy to convince yourself, if you have a really compelling plot. So you have to really, really be a good close reader and realize the amount of ambiguity. . . . We become a master, but we think we're more master than we are. There are plenty of other risks, too. It happens very rarely, but it happens that I just feel like I've crossed over a line and I'll say, "Oh, this lady needs a doctor." It happens rarely and it happens with or without these skills. But one has to keep taking the temperature of the relationship. . . . I think we have to pay attention to the risks. . . . I think there are internal risks to persons, even in our Narrative Medicine Workshops . . . there are some for whom this is too much and they kind of get in a little disarray. . . . I don't think persons should be armed with this set of "oh you can do this and do this and this" and be sent back in ill prepared for what's going to happen. That's what I mean, that's the risk. People start in on this kind of naively and then don't realize why suddenly they're feeling much sadder than they used to. Or suddenly they don't want any new patients anymore, or suddenly they are "jumpy" whenever their beeper goes off like they used to be as an intern.

JC: If you approach patients with a lack of flexibility and a determination to use only the tools that narrative-based medicine gives you, I think you do run a risk. It's quite clear that a large percentage of patients are not interested and don't come to the doctor with the kind of problems that allow you to make full use of these skills. There's also the practical risk. The practice of medicine is not structured in a way that allows you the time to do certain things that you might want to do. . . . In fact, it doesn't take a lot of time to establish connection with patients and to get an accurate picture of the patient narrative. It can be done in a short period of time. But this relates to the question of judgment, as to the nature of the patient's needs and wants, which determines the extent to which you're going to go. You've got to have a sense of how far you can use these skills in a given situation, or how much is warranted.

CD: There's a risk that a caregiver might direct the patient's narrative through questions that limit the telling or by using printed forms that direct the patient's responses. I mention this because in our hospital nurses have to fill out an 18-page admission form. I think this is a misguided attempt to evoke a patient narrative.

I think another risk is not including the patient in the interpretation of the narrative. For example, the patient tells her story. The caregiver listens. Then the caregiver interprets the narrative without considering the patient's interpretation. In that case there's a danger that "witnessing" could be replaced by an unconscious "controlling", particularly if the caregiver is a very concrete thinker who is not prone or trained to receive information metaphorically. Because patients so often speak in metaphor, if the provider is not aware of these subtleties, he or she might misinterpret the message behind the narrative. Sometimes the underbelly – the unspoken narrative – is more important than what is actually said.

I think there's a danger that narrative-based medicine might become just another "gimmick in the black bag", especially if it's forced upon students or practitioners who are resistant or who feel more drawn to the purely scientific, evidence-based way of practicing medicine or nursing. I think there's a danger that, because the time at the bedside is so limited, people may create tools to try and get at the narrative more quickly. Like the 18-page interview.

There's also some chance, particularly with a young caregiver, that a provider might be so carried away emotionally by the patient's narrative that he forgets to engage his intellect as well as his heart. He may not think of diagnosis and treatment because he's overwhelmed with emotion. I'm not sure this is a risk per se, but perhaps it is a stage that providers must go through when they begin truly listening to a patient's narrative.

Another possible risk in narrative-based medicine is if the goal becomes not the healing of the patient but the patient's story itself – especially in the academic arena. I have friends who are caregivers and also writers. Sometimes when they listen to patients' stories, they tell me, they're thinking "This would make a great poem" or "This would really be a good article." If this happens, then we may not attend quite as fully as we should be doing. As a writer, I often use my experiences with patients as a springboard for poems or stories. But these are usually interactions recollected when something else in the present triggers the memory. Then the two events come together in a way that results, I hope, in a work of literature that gives a more universal and metaphorical view of a particular caregiving event.

I think there's a danger, too, in our desire, and I include myself in this, to foster this academic genre we call narrative-based medicine or literature and medicine when what we're really talking about is simply listening attentively to what patients have to say. We can err on the side of becoming too regimented, making too many pronouncements about how to "do" narrative-based medicine or how to decide what it is and what it isn't. As a result, we may end up not allowing the patient narrative to flow quite as openly or easily as we say we want it to.

Narrative-based medicine, in my own experience, can also falter in the face of cultural differences. For example, in the clinic many of our patients don't speak English. I'm fairly fluent in Spanish, but for several years I was unaware of some of the more subtle cultural and linguistic issues. I was listening, but I was missing the important nuances of what patients were telling me.

TB: I think that sometimes it can distract you. I used to talk a lot about how I think we over-rely . . . on numbers and technology. Sometimes your patient's story is just so fascinating it can sort of take you aside, yet I wouldn't use it as a substitute for numbers and technology. It can be so deep sometimes, that you get distracted. I think the story is far more explanative, yet you can't see more than so many patients a day and really spend time and use a good narrative-based approach. I know some practitioners who see 50 patients in a day. You can't use narrative medicine and be profitable. That's where the risk is. If volume is important, you have to compromise somewhere.

CONDITIONS THAT HAVE PROMPTED A NARRATIVE MOVEMENT
I: What do you think currently divides caregivers from their patients?
VG: Cost and time, both of those pieces. The medicalization of issues so that for people to get relieved of some jobs, for example, the only way they can do that legitimately is to have a medical reason. I think there's also a social barrier because most physicians are highly educated and a lesser number of patients are. Even though I try to use language that's understandable and try to act in an approachable way, there always is a barrier there between the life that I live and know and the assumptions I make [for example] about having enough food to eat . . . having a home that's safe; having a life that's worth living . . . may not be the same assumptions for my patient.

RC: Heavens, so much divides us. . . . I'm well, you're sick. I'm rich, you're poor. I speak English, you don't. . . . You want a colonoscopy, I'm not going to authorize a colonoscopy unless you've done X, Y, and Z. . . . You want brand name Lipitor, you're only going to get Atorvastatin from me . . . up and down the line, horrible! It's this kind of stinginess.

. . . You know what it's coupled with? Greed. It's stinginess to our patients and I hate to say a lot of my colleagues are powered by greed! They will be damned if they don't make a certain amount of take-home profit from every day in practice. So they can't take Medicaid patients. They can only take Medicare, only if their patient pays the overcharge and down the line. A more sinister kind of greed, because it looks so healthy, is the "I want balance in my life." . . . But it's like come on . . . you do this work with one hand tied behind your back. . . . That's a kind of greed.

. . . Just the notion of "How much time do I have for you?" That's part of the greed and the stinginess. It's a chasm. It's alarming. It's horrible. It eats people up. We also have to pay attention to what divides us from one another. The doctor–nurse business is horrible.

JC: We live in a society where typically people don't listen to one another and don't take the time to observe situations carefully. Certainly they don't pay a lot of attention to the idea of developing empathic connections, except for maybe a small group of friends. We blame this on technology or blame it on the fast pace that we have. Medicine exists in a culture. And so our trainees come in, and they're put into a culture of medicine that reflects the overall culture. So there's very little priority put on the skills and techniques that are necessary to develop an empathic connection, especially to do it in a professional way.

The culture says what is important – the MRI scan, getting to the bottom of things, the disease, the defect, the problem is something that needs to be identified and removed. That's not a narrative way of looking at it. But that's what really divides caregivers from their patients.

CD: . . . I'll read you my long list: technology; more forms; better science and therefore more tests and machines and more forms; less need for physical exams because of the technology, therefore less intimacy between the patient and the caregiver, less laying on of hands, which can be both investigative and healing; managed care and insurance regulations that demand that we spend less time per patient; budget crunches.

The widening rift between management and clinicians. In many hospitals, the management tends to consist of young, business-oriented, very high-tech, high-stress, and high-energy people who often make decisions without including the clinical staff.

Terrible burnout among nurses and physicians; the belief on the part of many young doctors and nurses that medicine is a nine to five job and not a lifetime sacrifice or endeavor.

The advent of "hospitalists", which means patients won't have their primary care providers, and instead may see an unfamiliar doctor every 12 hours.

I think there's also been a major shift in the public image of both nurses and doctors. This may sound old fashioned, but nurses nowadays wear scrubs, sneakers, and are not required to tie up long hair, as we once were. Nurses just don't look as professional as they once did, and I think that's changed the public image of nursing. We aren't seen now as "angels in white." We've become women and men who run around, hair flying, wearing sneakers because we have to run so fast. Nurses don't have time to do what they once did – tend and know the patients . . .

In the past, physicians and nurses didn't mind staying late or seeing a patient in the evening – they didn't mind going that extra mile. Now providers know that if they do that, they're going to lose the hospital money. They're going to be overwhelmed. They're going to be denied overtime or at least reprimanded for working overtime and thus straining the budget. Perhaps this is another reason caregivers lean toward narrative-based medicine, in a way returning to a different set of values and a different way of doing things.

Some young caregivers are so afraid that if they open their hearts to patients and really develop "suffering hearts" or become "benevolent witnesses" they're going to be destroyed, both by their emotions and by all the other demands placed upon them today. I see this often in the new residents. If they really do open their hearts to patients and then suffer emotionally – both because they've gotten so close and because they can be chastised for "spending too much time" – then they might close down. They might retreat into the traditional pattern of getting in there, getting the facts, figuring out what's wrong, making a treatment decision, and then moving on. This is how they survive. The pressures to be efficient and to see a lot of patients are barriers to good care.

TB: The biggest thing that's dividing us . . . is third-party intermediaries, such as the government and insurance companies, who are empowered to have a larger say in what we do and how we do it. We also allow societal demand to dictate our actions – order more tests, prescribe newer medicines, and perform newer procedures, none of which are necessarily better. Unfortunately, getting involved in self-promotion in order to gain a market share also gets in the way of the fundamentals. Electronic Medical Records can also divide us from our patients, by encouraging template-driven documentation, which does not lend itself at all to emotion or narration. Government expects more documentation and objectivity. The insurance companies are moving toward people using that to determine payments. . . . Everybody wants technology, everybody wants the objective results. I think it really has been overemphasized and that to me is what divides our relationships. It is this tendency to drift and rely on the black and white – technology, tests, drugs. Everyone wants the drugs – everyone wants a pill to get better. "I can't sleep at night." "Well, why don't we talk about why you're not sleeping?" "I don't want to talk about it. I just want to ignore it." I think that's what's driving us apart.

EM: I think it's role perception. . . . The doctors think that they need to be an authority; they can't be human. The essence of relationship is the humanity that we all share. If you deny that or if you believe that you're placed in a role where you're not allowed to be a human being, that you're supposed to be an authority here and you're supposed to have the answers and you're responsible for this person's well-being, it's a very precarious position. It's very unsettling for people to be in it. They get very defensive.

JS: I think the main barrier is time. As a nurse or any caregiver, you feel a certain amount of "leading a patient on" if you only have two minutes. . . . You start asking questions which you know you don't have time to listen to. I think that's a frustration and a barrier. . . . It's very difficult to get the story when you have electronic charts. I know everybody thinks this is the best thing since sliced bread, but I'm not so sure.

THE RELATIONSHIP BETWEEN NARRATIVE MEDICINE AND OTHER RELATED MOVEMENTS

I: How do you see the relationship between narrative medicine, relationship-centered care, evidenced-based medicine, and professionalism?

VG: First of all, relationship-centered care. I immediately flashed to Gale Steven's diagram of the overlapping circles. One circle is the patient, one circle is the doctor, and the area of overlap is the doctor–patient relationship, which is relationship-centered care, in my mind. I think what narrative does is it helps increase that overlap. I think it facilitates that relationship. . . . It's hard to imagine having, in a sense, one without the other. It's hard for me to imagine practicing good relationship-centered care and not knowing the patient's narrative and the patient knowing some of my narrative, hopefully the amount that's appropriate for their needs . . .

Evidence-based medicine, of course, is an outcome of traditional understanding of what constitutes evidence within biomedicine, which dominates the professional assessment of what's good for the patient, what would be financed right now. Although certainly even the people like Trish Greenhalgh who promoted this would say that's only part of it. Certainly that's how most of us teach evidence-based medicine now. We have a responsibility to patients to bring them materials and information about what works. But whether it works in that particular patient, at that particular time, is less well known. Whether the patient chooses to have that particular . . . drug "X" that only works for 1 out of 10 patients. . . . It's the patient who makes the decision about whether they want to gamble and try and be that 1 in 10. Evidence-based medicine is a professional story, a professional "lens", and can be brought into the story of the relationship.

RC: I think it's important to bring these things together [narrative medicine and relationship-centered care] . . . when I talked to Tom Inui, Rich Frankel, Ron Epstein . . . and Tony Suchman . . . I said "Look, we're all in the same federation, we're different city/states. I'm narrative medicine; you're relationship-centered care. Ron, you're mindful practice. Moira Steward and her group are patient-centered." These are all city/states within a federation. As soon as we can name the federation, we're golden. It's something like effective health care or something. . . . I think it's relationship-centered care, patient-centered care, mindful practice, narrative medicine – at least those four. There may be more. . . . But you see how at least those four . . . are . . . "neighboring" concepts, sharing different things. . . . They're not identical, but they're highly, highly integrated.

Now, evidence-based, we've talked about a little bit. I just can't tell you how excited I am with this NEBM, narrative-evidence-based medicine because we keep saying, "Hey guys, what counts as evidence? Does the story count?" . . . They keep saying "Well, we know our evidence, but we can't marshal it for the sake of a given person, until we know something more about that person. How do we learn that?" . . . So that one, evidence-based, doesn't belong on this list. It's not in the federation exactly. . . . The real practitioners of evidence-based medicine realize that there are at least three integrating circles – one is the evidence itself from randomized clinical trials, one is patient preferences and values, and one is provider or clinician skills. These things have to be in concert.

. . . When you start talking about professionalism, students feel that you're blaming them . . . you're not doing (whatever it is) enough. . . . There are two words I've never known what to do with. One is professionalism. The other is humanism. . . . So, those two are words I don't use. . . . We just have to be on the alert for professionalism as, I think, a code word for "it's your fault."

JC: I think relationship-centered care or person-centered care deals with the same issues, and so it's closely related to narrative medicine. . . . Evidence-based medicine is a different movement. There may be some indirect relationship. But, basically, evidence-based medicine is trying to make medicine more scientific.

Again, it [professionalism] is an attempt to enhance the quality of physicians from a moral, ethical perspective as well as a relationship perspective. So again, I suppose, in a sense that is indirectly related to narrative-based medicine.

CD: I suppose there would have to be a relationship between relationship-centered care and narrative-based medicine, because narrative is all about "relationships."

I think that evidence-based medicine can sometimes, or often, discount the caregiver's individual intuition and experiences. Therefore it has the potential to defeat narrative-based interactions – evidence-based medicine might not accept much of the patient narrative as "fitting into" the evidence-based parameters. A patient might tell his or her story, but the provider thinks, well, that can't possibly be accurate because the "evidence" says something else. Evidence-based medicine tends to encourage providers to leap ahead of the patient's story and not allow the patient's story its fullness. It tends to discount not only the patient's story, but also a huge part of the caregiver's intuitive and instinctual feelings about what may be going on . . .

Unfortunately, I think we can be extremely professional and yet not be emotionally connected to the patient at all. So, in some ways, professionalism could be a hindrance to narrative-based medicine – if professionalism doesn't go hand in hand with emotional connection. The demands of "professionalism" might make providers think that they should take five steps back, fold their hands or put their hands in their pockets, nod, and then, after they've politely listened, sit down and say "This is what I think." Again, it depends totally on the individual caregiver. Can you teach professionalism? I don't know. I think professionalism is like intuition or true compassion. We can make providers aware and we can encourage professionalism – but in the end you either have it or you don't.

REACTIONS TO SOME FREQUENTLY MENTIONED ISSUES ASSOCIATED WITH NARRATIVE PRACTICE

I: It has been said that illness stories are about disruptions in a patient's life trajectory. Do you see it that way? What is the nature of these disruptions? Does the clinician have a responsibility to restore coherence to the illness story?

VG: I think what we struggle with is [that] illness stories are about disruptions in a patient's life trajectory. The job of the physician and the patient is to work so there is coherence and not disruption so the illness is not disrupting the patient's life, but that the illness is part of the patient's life so that you work through it. I forget where I read [that] people think that life shouldn't have any suffering. But suffering is part of life. . . . How can I be whole with suffering as part of my life? How can I incorporate the suffering into part of [me]? Not a destructive me, but just a part of me.

RC: Everything meaningful is disrupted. No, we do not have a responsibility to restore coherence, absolutely not. That's master–slave business. We have the opportunity to let a person hear him- or herself tell it. In the telling, if there's a restoration of coherence, it's from the person telling. . . . There are times when, from the vantage point of a skilled listener, we can kind of hear a linkage that the person telling it doesn't. When I say to the person, "I'm glad your joints are feeling better, how are things at home?" . . . that's an example of seeing something that might help you connect these bits, but that's as far as I think we can go with that. I like the idea of disruptions. There's a lot of literary critical work about disruptions. If there are no disruptions, you're dead!

I think we get too wedded to the imagery of the trajectory. These are not elliptical paths of orbit. . . . It's not like you graduate from college then you plot it all out. I think we get carried away with our sense of orderliness and linear plot.

JC: Well, it's hard to say. What is a life trajectory? It's part of a patient's story. We're just selecting out parts of the current story or the story that the patient chooses, a problem to come to the doctor with. So I don't like to think that illness stories are disruptions in a life trajectory. There is no platonic archetype of a person's life trajectory. Whatever happens to you is your life trajectory, and illness is a part of that. Illness is natural. . . . I don't think there's anything incoherent about an illness story. I guess it's only incoherent in the sense that it doesn't fit in, it's not understood. So it's the physician's responsibility to help resolve illness, or more often to help the patient understand the illness and learn to live with it. If you want to interpret that as restoring coherence to a story, I guess you could say that.

CD: I really see illness not as a disruption but as a continuation of a particular life. The time of illness is just as significant as the "real" life that went before or that may come after. It's difficult for patients and caregivers to accept that. I very much feel that illness and health are both part of your life.

I don't believe that the caregiver has any responsibility to restore coherence to the patient's illness story. I think the patient may achieve a certain amount of coherence through the telling of his or her illness story. That coherence may only consist of the ability to accept the current chaos and to exist within it – perhaps nothing more than that, but that would be quite an achievement.

Of course, I think the caregiver has a responsibility to do whatever he or she can to help the patient, but that help has to be the help that the patient wants, whether that means pain relief or cure, palliation or assistance to transfer into a dying process. I don't think caregivers can restore coherence to the patient's experience. I think if we try to do that, we're really trying to restore our own coherence, not the patient's. We have to accept that our patients are who they are at the time of their sickness, and then we have to do the best we can to be with them.

EM: I spoke to one of my patients last week or the week before who had metastatic lymph cancer. He'd just found out about it three days before. . . . I had seen him six months ago and he was healthy. . . . He'd had a lot of problems along the way, a lot of heart issues. The heart issues were resolved. He was doing fine from that perspective. Now he was looking ahead at a lot of chemo. . . . He just said, "I'm going to take it as it comes." For him, it was a minor disruption. I think he had practice at this before from overcoming these physical obstacles with his heart. He felt like he was on borrowed time anyway because any one of those things before should have done him in. He now had something that was going to be a struggle that was probably what he was going to die of. He was OK with it. His life trajectory really had been interrupted before. . . . The reason he talked about it with me was because we'd talked about everything before. He was one of the patients I'd known for five or six years. It was very concerning for him. He was worried about his wife. We talked about that.

JS: If you would've asked me that question 20 years ago, I would say "absolutely it's a disruption." Now I would say everybody's story evolves, like a journey. Just because you're ill or you go through an illness doesn't mean you're not whole. It simply becomes part of your experience, so your story changes. It becomes a different story and a richer story.

I: What will it take for narrative health care to become firmly established, to become part of routine practice and not just a current fad? What are the barriers to this happening?
VG: . . . it's the time issue that's a big issue, and I worry about just taking snippets of patients' stories, counting it as a whole in order to deal with the time, then it becomes fallacious.

RC: Oh boy, it's going to take lots of legislative work, isn't it? The pharmaceutical industry and the insurance industry are going to have to be banished. That's saying a lot. I think we can do it. I think that some of the [upcoming] electoral politics are going to help. I think it is within 10 years that we'll have universal health care. . . . It's going to take a great deal of legislative power and some major changes in our own democracy. So this is not something medicine can do by itself.

. . . If you think just in the past two or three years of what we've learned about narrative medicine, you're amazed. If you include the whole federation, it's major. . . . Whole generations of medical students are being trained different ways. The inter-health profession, the doctor–nurse–social worker stuff, is really, really taking off. We're teaching the physical therapists, the occupational therapists, the pastoral care interns, the social workers. It's thrilling. . . . Each thing that divides us, I think we're getting some grasp on. I end up feeling just so amazingly, blissfully optimistic.

JC: There are many barriers, but most important is the culture we live in. In so far as our approach to medicine is counter-cultural, we're going to be facing an uphill battle, not only from health insurers and hospitals, etc., but also from patients. . . . Patients would be a barrier if they want medicine that is based primarily on diagnostic tests and technical intervention. If those things are inappropriate and you are trying to develop a narrative interaction with them to assist them, but this is different from what they expect, then you have to modify their expectations. In that sense, patients could be a barrier. Most physicians will tell you that it is much more difficult to engage people in stories, or to teach them about probability, than it is to simply order an MRI.

CD: I think that for narrative-based medicine to become firmly established, it would take a miracle. We'd have to have a whole lot more time to spend with patients. We'd have to use less forms, which means the state and the insurance companies would be very unhappy with how we were documenting. We'd have to educate students differently. We'd have to educate patients, who are not used to a narrative-based approach anymore. We'd have to re-educate hospital administrations to focus less on the "bottom line" and more on patient satisfaction – but of course if patient satisfaction increased it would help the bottom line. We'd have to hire a lot more nurses. We're very concerned today about errors and medical mistakes, but the very forms and rituals that we put in place to limit these mistakes sometimes contribute to the mistakes. Narrative-based medicine will only become firmly established when everyone sees value in returning to the bedside. Unfortunately, in today's managed care environment, the bottom line rules.

. . . One of my concerns is that narrative-based medicine has become an interesting intellectual and cultural pursuit – but that this interest fades when students graduate. Fortunately, there are many practitioners – both physicians and nurses – who do believe that paying attention to narrative is the best way to interact with patients, both for the patient's sake and for the caregiver's. This small group keeps the concept of narrative-based medicine alive. But if this small group is in academia and not engaged with patients at the bedside, then the concept of narrative-based medicine is being sustained, but not the actual practice.

For now, maybe all we can do is to recognize those caregivers who have that "spark", that intuition, the ability to be a benevolent witness, a suffering heart, and to encourage them. To tell them it's okay for them to use those attributes in their practice. To tell them that it's okay to sit down and listen to a patient. I just don't see narrative-based healthcare ever becoming firmly established. It's limited not by the ideals of narrative-based medicine but by the reality of how we "do" healthcare today, and by individual practitioners who are not capable of or who don't see the value in narrative-based care. There may be barriers on the patient's side, too. Some patients don't want to reveal their narrative, just as some caregivers don't want to hear it.

TB: . . . I don't see a single force . . . other than those of us talking about it, and those writing about it. That's moving us in that direction. The government is the force; the insurance company is the force. There's no CPT code for conversation. Everything is numbers. What would it take? We have to un-do the current system or at least talk about it. . . . Take a capable internist who wants a limited practice, to see a finite number of patients. If he gives each and every one of them the real time they deserve in real face time, real one-on-one time, real routine follow-ups, real emergency availability, he's not going to be allowed to do it. The government is fighting it. Insurance companies are fighting it. Nobody wants that to happen. . . . You almost have to go back to a one-on-one relationship, eliminate third parties, then individual control would be preserved. The patients would look for the proper care with doctors who saw them as the individuals they are, and who provided care in keeping with their perspective, desires, and beliefs. You've got doctors who would provide that mutually beneficial relationship, but as long as you have a third party, whether it be the government or [an insurance company], it gets to be a tremendous barrier. It's not all black and white. It's all gray out there. How do you convince people we want to get away from black and white, and we want to go back to gray?

EM: . . . I've worked with some great [nurses], who take time with their patients. That's the key. . . . There's time pressure, reimbursement pressure, that's what's going to hold narrative-based medicine back, because it's a time-consuming thing. You can do really good work, over time. You're seeing the same patient and you don't have to "re-invent the wheel." You jump into your relationship with them. They tell you what's going on. It can be a really quick thing. . . . They get educated really fast. . . . For me, the key is the extra time that you are allowed to spend.

Afterword

I am a 52-year-old white male family physician celebrating the 25th anniversary of becoming John Engel's friend and colleague, and am grateful to him for introducing me to the other wonderful people who have contributed to this remarkable book. It is an enormous privilege to share in this Afterword my thoughts about the book and about the issues that it touches upon.

Health care has a broken heart. Chapter 1 opens with a quote from Bernard Lown: ". . . the doctor, by virtue of accepting science so totally, creates a total imbalance, forgetting the art of healing, forgetting the art of engagement, forgetting the art of listening, forgetting the art of caring and ceasing to invest time with the patient. So I believe that medicine has lost its human face." What he says is true, but "accepting science so totally" is only one of the reasons for the problem. A few years ago, I took some time to interview graduates of the Virginia Commonwealth University – Blackstone Family Medicine Residency Program, whose mission was to produce family physicians for rural Virginia. Many of the graduates told me how overwhelmed they felt in the face of inadequate access to primary care in the communities that they served with great dedication. They were taught to incorporate careful listening to their patients and to spend adequate time with them, but felt forced to abandon this model in the face of having to see 40 or more patients every day – not to make adequate income, but because they *had to* in order to meet the acute, chronic, and preventive health care needs of their community. One of them summed it up as follows: "I can't practice medicine the way I was taught at Blackstone." So the sheer inadequacy of some of the critical parts of our health care system is a "root cause" for a willing but broken heart in many caregivers.

Another source of the tenacious grip of reductionism is that the attendant move to specialization has enormous economic incentives behind it, at least in the US system. This power is very hard to resist – we have created one of the major economic engines for our country with our "health care–industrial complex." Each year, we spend US$ 2 trillion on health care, and achieve relatively poor results compared with other industrialized nations. Yet the resistance to change is enormous (remember Hillary Clinton's efforts in the

1990s) – one person's waste is another person's income! The author of Chapter 2 seems to hint at this dynamic in talking about the cultural and economic pressures for "soft" disciplines to become more procedure-based. Rita Charon acknowledges this directly in her interview portrayed in Chapter 8, where she speaks about the shameful greed of some of her colleagues, and it is certainly another root cause of health care's broken heart.

Reductionism and specialization, as the authors point out, are fully evident in the curricula of our medical schools, and the training of other health care professionals. The authors of this book and the other leaders of the humanist movement struggle to introduce ways of thinking and being that sadly seem foreign and out of place. In medicine, for example, the typical experience of students is metaphorically described as "drinking from a fire hose." So we try to create antidotes to the insanely overpacked curriculum that has an inordinate emphasis on basic science knowledge that most of the graduates will never remember, and will never use when they are caring for their patients. In trying to re-introduce humanism into the medical school curriculum, are we guilty of a kind of "poly-curriculum" – giving another curricular "medication" to counteract the "side effects" of a dehumanizing way of teaching? In the face of a call by the Association of American Medical Colleges (AAMC) to train 30% more physicians, and with new medical schools springing up all over the country, I see an opportunity for thoughtful medical educators to create another model of training physicians that is far more practical, that preserves and grows the innate humanism of our matriculants, that is far less expensive than our current profligate curricula, and that takes the Hippocratic oath's pledge to patients of "first, do no harm" and makes that same promise to our medical students. Can't those creating new schools say "We can do so much better than merely copying the status quo"? In the case of patient care, the Institute for Healthcare Improvement now crystallizes its mission as a "triple aim" of reduced overall costs of care, superior patient experience of care, and superior quality of care. Many innovative clinicians have demonstrated that it is possible to achieve all three at the same time. Surely we must have the same aim for how we educate future health care practitioners – reduced overall costs of education, superior student experience of education, and superior practitioners as our end product. I ask accrediting organizations, can you imagine accrediting new models that achieve this educational "triple aim"?

Charon and others who were interviewed for the final chapter sometimes sound despairing, and say that for humanism to be fully reintegrated into how health care is taught and practiced, it will take a broad restructuring of how it is financed and delivered. Take heart, Rita! There are organizations that have done just that for themselves – not waiting for state or national reforms. Learn about companies like QuadGraphics (www.qg.com; see also www.quad-med.com), where a self-insured financing model has primary care physicians spending half an hour with each patient yet receiving incomes that are better than those of their colleagues in "churn to earn" models of care, where employees overwhelmingly prefer the "company doctors" for their care, and where the company is saving tens of millions of dollars each year on health care costs. The heart of medicine must be beating strongly in these places.

While practice redesign creates new opportunities for a reintegration of narrative medicine, we also need to talk about personal redesign. So many primary care physicians, nurses, and other health care practitioners seem to be saying to their professional associations, "Fix my life." These are broken-hearted caregivers who feel victimized and powerless. It is very tempting for large professional associations to try to rescue them, but I believe that there is more power in each one of us who feels that way to rescue ourselves and to help our brother and sister caregivers to do the same. What if each of us committed to the following steps?

- Find a professional colleague we trust, and ask them to "hold up a mirror" to us.*
- Look in the mirror.
- See and celebrate the goodness.
- See and forgive the flaws.
- Accept that some suffering in our professional lives is inevitable, and reframe it as an opportunity for personal growth (as the authors of this book point out, that is precisely what we try to help our patients to do when they are suffering).
- Learn that some suffering is self-created and that it *can* be eliminated (the ideas of the Serenity Prayer are precisely applicable here).
- Invest in relationships with colleagues – share meals on a regular basis, listen and care, and don't try to "fix their lives!"

What if we have the courage to walk away from "hamster-wheel medicine"?† What if we consciously integrate personal redesign with practice redesign (and throw in some regular attention to political advocacy)?

> Two roads diverged in a wood, and I –
> I took the one less traveled by,
> And that has made all the difference.

> *Robert Frost*

Narrative medicine is, to the detriment of too many patients, currently the road less traveled. Let us instead make it the path of choice – that will make all the difference to those we serve.

Anton J Kuzel MD, MHPE

---

* David Marsland MD, personal communication.

† Joseph Scherger MD, personal communication.

Glossary

Affective. Pertaining to feeling and emotion.

Blunting Affect. Purposefully or subconsciously dampening or burying feelings and emotions.

Burnout. The breakdown of an individual emotionally and sometimes physically.

Cartesian Dualism. The theory that mind and body are independent and irreducible phenomena.

Clerkship. The clinical training process for medical students under the supervision of resident physicians and seasoned physician faculty in the hospital or medical office which generally occurs in the third year of medical school.

Cognitive. Relating to knowledge in the most general sense, or the ability of the mind to know.

Critical Social Theory. A blend of practical philosophy and explanatory social science. Practical philosophy deals with the particulars of moral and political life and the actions necessary to achieve a good life. Explanatory social science is concerned with changing social action.

Empathy. A process of exercising one's moral imagination to facilitate emotional resonance with patients.

Epistemological Dualism. The idea that the perception of an object is separate and distinct from the object itself.

Epistemology. The branch of philosophy that is concerned with the genesis, nature, structure, and legitimacy of knowledge. There are many competing theories of knowledge, with some being more privileged than others in any given historical period.

Ethnomethodology. This term was coined by the sociologist Harold Garfinkel. It is the study of how people, as reflective social actors, accomplish the actions of everyday life.

Existentialism. This is both a philosophical and literary movement, which originated in France following World War Two. In the social sciences, it was a reaction against a strong version of cognitive sociology that viewed the individual as separate and distinct from the production of knowledge.

Haiku. A Japanese poetry form most often consisting of three lines, the first and third lines having five syllables and the second line having seven syllables.

Hermeneutic. Referring to the theory, art, and philosophy of interpretation, and to deriving the meaning of events and phenomena in general.

Illness. The human experience of symptoms and suffering.

Mantra. A pattern of words, symbols, shapes, or pictures used to quiet the mind.

Mindfulness. The state of being closely attentive to another person; listening attentively and responding meaningfully.

Ontology. The branch of philosophy that is concerned with questions about existence and reality in the world.

Paradigm. A world view or general perspective along with a set of commitments, beliefs, values, and methods.

Phenomenology. First applied by Edmund Husserl, a philosophical position that emphasizes descriptive analyses of subjective processes to reach their underlying meanings.

Presence. The state of being present with another not only physically, but also emotionally and spiritually.

Principlist. A term coined by Howard Brody to describe an individual who adheres to the principles and traditionally delineated methods of deliberating ethical dilemmas.

Professionalization. The act of assimilating the culture of a profession, its customs, policies, procedures, etc.

Reflective Interior. The ability to reflect on or examine matters in the mind without necessarily talking about them.

Social Constructivism. The idea that humans do not find or discover knowledge so much as construct it. Knowledge is contingent on human perception and sociocultural experience bracketed by time.

Sympathy. The ability to join in the depth of the feelings of another person, or to assume the feelings of another person.

Teleological. Referring to the philosophical view that explains the past and present in terms of the future. It is contrasted with mechanistic views, which explain the present and the future in terms of the past. Referring to the view that the mind is governed by purposes, interests, and values.

Author index

Subject index